AMBIEN

A MEDICAL DICTIONARY, BIBLIOGRAPHY,
AND ANNOTATED RESEARCH GUIDE TO
INTERNET REFERENCES

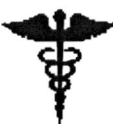

JAMES N. PARKER, M.D.
AND PHILIP M. PARKER, PH.D., EDITORS

ICON Health Publications
ICON Group International, Inc.
4370 La Jolla Village Drive, 4th Floor
San Diego, CA 92122 USA

Copyright ©2003 by ICON Group International, Inc.

Copyright ©2003 by ICON Group International, Inc. All rights reserved. This book is protected by copyright. No part of it may be reproduced, stored in a retrieval system, or transmitted in any form or by any means, electronic, mechanical, photocopying, recording, or otherwise, without written permission from the publisher.

Printed in the United States of America.

Last digit indicates print number: 10 9 8 7 6 4 5 3 2 1

Publisher, Health Care: Philip Parker, Ph.D.
Editor(s): James Parker, M.D., Philip Parker, Ph.D.

Publisher's note: The ideas, procedures, and suggestions contained in this book are not intended for the diagnosis or treatment of a health problem. As new medical or scientific information becomes available from academic and clinical research, recommended treatments and drug therapies may undergo changes. The authors, editors, and publisher have attempted to make the information in this book up to date and accurate in accord with accepted standards at the time of publication. The authors, editors, and publisher are not responsible for errors or omissions or for consequences from application of the book, and make no warranty, expressed or implied, in regard to the contents of this book. Any practice described in this book should be applied by the reader in accordance with professional standards of care used in regard to the unique circumstances that may apply in each situation. The reader is advised to always check product information (package inserts) for changes and new information regarding dosage and contraindications before prescribing any drug or pharmacological product. Caution is especially urged when using new or infrequently ordered drugs, herbal remedies, vitamins and supplements, alternative therapies, complementary therapies and medicines, and integrative medical treatments.

Cataloging-in-Publication Data

Parker, James N., 1961-
Parker, Philip M., 1960-

Ambien: A Medical Dictionary, Bibliography, and Annotated Research Guide to Internet References / James N. Parker and Philip M. Parker, editors
        p.   cm.
Includes bibliographical references, glossary, and index.
ISBN: 0-597-83693-0
1. Ambien-Popular works.   I. Title.

Disclaimer

This publication is not intended to be used for the diagnosis or treatment of a health problem. It is sold with the understanding that the publisher, editors, and authors are not engaging in the rendering of medical, psychological, financial, legal, or other professional services.

References to any entity, product, service, or source of information that may be contained in this publication should not be considered an endorsement, either direct or implied, by the publisher, editors, or authors. ICON Group International, Inc., the editors, and the authors are not responsible for the content of any Web pages or publications referenced in this publication.

Copyright Notice

If a physician wishes to copy limited passages from this book for patient use, this right is automatically granted without written permission from ICON Group International, Inc. (ICON Group). However, all of ICON Group publications have copyrights. With exception to the above, copying our publications in whole or in part, for whatever reason, is a violation of copyright laws and can lead to penalties and fines. Should you want to copy tables, graphs, or other materials, please contact us to request permission (E-mail: iconedit@san.rr.com). ICON Group often grants permission for very limited reproduction of our publications for internal use, press releases, and academic research. Such reproduction requires confirmed permission from ICON Group International Inc. **The disclaimer above must accompany all reproductions, in whole or in part, of this book.**

Acknowledgements

The collective knowledge generated from academic and applied research summarized in various references has been critical in the creation of this book which is best viewed as a comprehensive compilation and collection of information prepared by various official agencies which produce publications on Ambien. Books in this series draw from various agencies and institutions associated with the United States Department of Health and Human Services, and in particular, the Office of the Secretary of Health and Human Services (OS), the Administration for Children and Families (ACF), the Administration on Aging (AOA), the Agency for Healthcare Research and Quality (AHRQ), the Agency for Toxic Substances and Disease Registry (ATSDR), the Centers for Disease Control and Prevention (CDC), the Food and Drug Administration (FDA), the Healthcare Financing Administration (HCFA), the Health Resources and Services Administration (HRSA), the Indian Health Service (IHS), the institutions of the National Institutes of Health (NIH), the Program Support Center (PSC), and the Substance Abuse and Mental Health Services Administration (SAMHSA). In addition to these sources, information gathered from the National Library of Medicine, the United States Patent Office, the European Union, and their related organizations has been invaluable in the creation of this book. Some of the work represented was financially supported by the Research and Development Committee at INSEAD. This support is gratefully acknowledged. Finally, special thanks are owed to Tiffany Freeman for her excellent editorial support.

About the Editors

James N. Parker, M.D.

Dr. James N. Parker received his Bachelor of Science degree in Psychobiology from the University of California, Riverside and his M.D. from the University of California, San Diego. In addition to authoring numerous research publications, he has lectured at various academic institutions. Dr. Parker is the medical editor for health books by ICON Health Publications.

Philip M. Parker, Ph.D.

Philip M. Parker is the Eli Lilly Chair Professor of Innovation, Business and Society at INSEAD (Fontainebleau, France and Singapore). Dr. Parker has also been Professor at the University of California, San Diego and has taught courses at Harvard University, the Hong Kong University of Science and Technology, the Massachusetts Institute of Technology, Stanford University, and UCLA. Dr. Parker is the associate editor for ICON Health Publications.

About ICON Health Publications

To discover more about ICON Health Publications, simply check with your preferred online booksellers, including Barnes & Noble.com and Amazon.com which currently carry all of our titles. Or, feel free to contact us directly for bulk purchases or institutional discounts:

>ICON Group International, Inc.
>4370 La Jolla Village Drive, Fourth Floor
>San Diego, CA 92122 USA
>Fax: 858-546-4341
>Web site: **www.icongrouponline.com/health**

Table of Contents

FORWARD	1
CHAPTER 1. STUDIES ON AMBIEN	3
Overview	3
The Combined Health Information Database	3
Federally Funded Research on Ambien	4
E-Journals: PubMed Central	5
The National Library of Medicine: PubMed	5
CHAPTER 2. NUTRITION AND AMBIEN	21
Overview	21
Finding Nutrition Studies on Ambien	21
Federal Resources on Nutrition	24
Additional Web Resources	25
CHAPTER 3. ALTERNATIVE MEDICINE AND AMBIEN	27
Overview	27
National Center for Complementary and Alternative Medicine	27
Additional Web Resources	28
General References	30
CHAPTER 4. PATENTS ON AMBIEN	31
Overview	31
Patents on Ambien	31
Patent Applications on Ambien	33
Keeping Current	34
CHAPTER 5. PERIODICALS AND NEWS ON AMBIEN	35
Overview	35
News Services and Press Releases	35
Academic Periodicals covering Ambien	37
CHAPTER 6. RESEARCHING MEDICATIONS	39
Overview	39
U.S. Pharmacopeia	39
Commercial Databases	40
Researching Orphan Drugs	40
APPENDIX A. PHYSICIAN RESOURCES	45
Overview	45
NIH Guidelines	45
NIH Databases	47
Other Commercial Databases	49
APPENDIX B. PATIENT RESOURCES	51
Overview	51
Patient Guideline Sources	51
Finding Associations	53
APPENDIX C. FINDING MEDICAL LIBRARIES	55
Overview	55
Preparation	55
Finding a Local Medical Library	55
Medical Libraries in the U.S. and Canada	55
ONLINE GLOSSARIES	61
Online Dictionary Directories	61
AMBIEN DICTIONARY	63

INDEX **83**

FORWARD

In March 2001, the National Institutes of Health issued the following warning: "The number of Web sites offering health-related resources grows every day. Many sites provide valuable information, while others may have information that is unreliable or misleading."[1] Furthermore, because of the rapid increase in Internet-based information, many hours can be wasted searching, selecting, and printing. Since only the smallest fraction of information dealing with Ambien is indexed in search engines, such as **www.google.com** or others, a non-systematic approach to Internet research can be not only time consuming, but also incomplete. This book was created for medical professionals, students, and members of the general public who want to know as much as possible about Ambien, using the most advanced research tools available and spending the least amount of time doing so.

In addition to offering a structured and comprehensive bibliography, the pages that follow will tell you where and how to find reliable information covering virtually all topics related to Ambien, from the essentials to the most advanced areas of research. Public, academic, government, and peer-reviewed research studies are emphasized. Various abstracts are reproduced to give you some of the latest official information available to date on Ambien. Abundant guidance is given on how to obtain free-of-charge primary research results via the Internet. **While this book focuses on the field of medicine, when some sources provide access to non-medical information relating to Ambien, these are noted in the text.**

E-book and electronic versions of this book are fully interactive with each of the Internet sites mentioned (clicking on a hyperlink automatically opens your browser to the site indicated). If you are using the hard copy version of this book, you can access a cited Web site by typing the provided Web address directly into your Internet browser. You may find it useful to refer to synonyms or related terms when accessing these Internet databases. **NOTE:** At the time of publication, the Web addresses were functional. However, some links may fail due to URL address changes, which is a common occurrence on the Internet.

For readers unfamiliar with the Internet, detailed instructions are offered on how to access electronic resources. For readers unfamiliar with medical terminology, a comprehensive glossary is provided. For readers without access to Internet resources, a directory of medical libraries, that have or can locate references cited here, is given. We hope these resources will prove useful to the widest possible audience seeking information on Ambien.

The Editors

---

[1] From the NIH, National Cancer Institute (NCI): **http://www.cancer.gov/cancerinfo/ten-things-to-know**.

CHAPTER 1. STUDIES ON AMBIEN

Overview

In this chapter, we will show you how to locate peer-reviewed references and studies on Ambien.

The Combined Health Information Database

The Combined Health Information Database summarizes studies across numerous federal agencies. To limit your investigation to research studies and Ambien, you will need to use the advanced search options. First, go to **http://chid.nih.gov/index.html**. From there, select the "Detailed Search" option (or go directly to that page with the following hyperlink: **http://chid.nih.gov/detail/detail.html**). The trick in extracting studies is found in the drop boxes at the bottom of the search page where "You may refine your search by." Select the dates and language you prefer, and the format option "Journal Article." At the top of the search form, select the number of records you would like to see (we recommend 100) and check the box to display "whole records." We recommend that you type "Ambien" (or synonyms) into the "For these words:" box. Consider using the option "anywhere in record" to make your search as broad as possible. If you want to limit the search to only a particular field, such as the title of the journal, then select this option in the "Search in these fields" drop box. The following is what you can expect from this type of search:

- **Sleep Disorders: A Common Problem Among Kidney Patients?**

    Source: For Patients Only. 8(1): 8-10, 24. January-February 1995.

    Contact: Available from Contemporary Dialysis, Inc. 6300 Variel Avenue, Suite I, Woodland Hills, CA 91367.

    Summary: In this article, the author provides readers with information about an often-encountered, but little-discussed complication of dialysis, insomnia. Topics include the adequacy of dialysis and its impact on the sleep habits of patients; restless leg syndrome (RLS) and the role of peripheral neuropathy in its development; the use of Sinemet to treat RLS; using conventional sleep aids, including **Ambien;** the use of muscle relaxants, or benzodiazepines, for milder forms of RLS; psychological sleep disturbances; and adjunctive therapies, including Qigong, biofeedback, and meditation. The author encourages readers to become more self-aware and to participate as an active member of their own health care team. The article includes a short list of references and organizations that may provide additional information about sleep disorders and their therapy.

Federally Funded Research on Ambien

The U.S. Government supports a variety of research studies relating to Ambien. These studies are tracked by the Office of Extramural Research at the National Institutes of Health.[2] CRISP (Computerized Retrieval of Information on Scientific Projects) is a searchable database of federally funded biomedical research projects conducted at universities, hospitals, and other institutions.

Search the CRISP Web site at **http://crisp.cit.nih.gov/crisp/crisp_query.generate_screen**. You will have the option to perform targeted searches by various criteria, including geography, date, and topics related to Ambien.

For most of the studies, the agencies reporting into CRISP provide summaries or abstracts. As opposed to clinical trial research using patients, many federally funded studies use animals or simulated models to explore Ambien. The following is typical of the type of information found when searching the CRISP database for Ambien:

- **Project Title: DISTINCTIVE INTEROCEPTIVE EFFECTS OF ALPHA 1 SELECTIVE GABA MODULATOR ZOLPIDEM**

    Principal Investigator & Institution: Rowlett, James K.; Harvard University (Medical School) Medical School Campus Boston, Ma 02115

    Timing: Fiscal Year 2001

    Summary: Zolpidem (Ambien) is a commonly prescribed sleep-aid that exhibits selectivity for benzodiazepine (BZ)/GABAA receptors containing the alpha-1 subunit Previous studies have suggested that **zolpidem** has a characteristic profile of subjective effects that differ from those of conventional BZ agonists The present study assessed the ability of BZs and barbiturates, which typically share interoceptive effects with BZs, to reproduce the effects of **zolpidem** in squirrel monkeys trained to discriminate **zolpidem** from vehicle The effects of **zolpidem** also were assessed in squirrel monkeys trained to discriminate another sleep-aid, triazolam (Halcion) Under test conditions, **zolpidem** engendered a dose-dependent increase in zolpidem-lever responding, reaching an average maximum of r80% Triazolam and diazepam also engendered r80% zolpidem-lever responding However, other BZ agonists including chlordiazepoxide and lorazepam, as well as the barbiturates pentobarbital, bar bital, and methohexital, engendered maximums of only 20-70% zolpidem-lever responding up to doses that markedly reduced response rate In contrast, **zolpidem,** chlordiazepoxide and lorazepam substituted fully in monkeys trained to discriminate triazolam using a similar procedure These results suggest that zolpidem's selectivity for the alpha-1 subunit of the BZ/GABAA receptor complex confers a profile of interoceptive effects that is unique compared to typical BZ agonists

---

[2] Healthcare projects are funded by the National Institutes of Health (NIH), Substance Abuse and Mental Health Services (SAMHSA), Health Resources and Services Administration (HRSA), Food and Drug Administration (FDA), Centers for Disease Control and Prevention (CDCP), Agency for Healthcare Research and Quality (AHRQ), and Office of Assistant Secretary of Health (OASH).

Website: http://crisp.cit.nih.gov/crisp/Crisp_Query.Generate_Screen

E-Journals: PubMed Central[3]

PubMed Central (PMC) is a digital archive of life sciences journal literature developed and managed by the National Center for Biotechnology Information (NCBI) at the U.S. National Library of Medicine (NLM).[4] Access to this growing archive of e-journals is free and unrestricted.[5] To search, go to **http://www.ncbi.nlm.nih.gov/entrez/query.fcgi?db=Pmc**, and type "Ambien" (or synonyms) into the search box. This search gives you access to full-text articles. The following is a sample of items found for Ambien in the PubMed Central database:

- **Hepatotoxicity associated with zolpidem treatment.** by Karsenti D, Blanc P, Bacq Y, Metman EH.; 1999 May 1; http://www.pubmedcentral.gov/articlerender.fcgi?tool=pmcentrez&artid=27854

The National Library of Medicine: PubMed

One of the quickest and most comprehensive ways to find academic studies in both English and other languages is to use PubMed, maintained by the National Library of Medicine.[6] The advantage of PubMed over previously mentioned sources is that it covers a greater number of domestic and foreign references. It is also free to use. If the publisher has a Web site that offers full text of its journals, PubMed will provide links to that site, as well as to sites offering other related data. User registration, a subscription fee, or some other type of fee may be required to access the full text of articles in some journals.

To generate your own bibliography of studies dealing with Ambien, simply go to the PubMed Web site at **http://www.ncbi.nlm.nih.gov/pubmed**. Type "Ambien" (or synonyms) into the search box, and click "Go." The following is the type of output you can expect from PubMed for Ambien (hyperlinks lead to article summaries):

- **A comparison of the residual effects of zaleplon and zolpidem following administration 5 to 2 h before awakening.**
  Author(s): Danjou P, Paty I, Fruncillo R, Worthington P, Unruh M, Cevallos W, Martin P.
  Source: British Journal of Clinical Pharmacology. 1999 September; 48(3): 367-74.
  http://www.ncbi.nlm.nih.gov:80/entrez/query.fcgi?cmd=Retrieve&db=PubMed&list_uids=10510148&dopt=Abstract

---

[3] Adapted from the National Library of Medicine: **http://www.pubmedcentral.nih.gov/about/intro.html**.

[4] With PubMed Central, NCBI is taking the lead in preservation and maintenance of open access to electronic literature, just as NLM has done for decades with printed biomedical literature. PubMed Central aims to become a world-class library of the digital age.

[5] The value of PubMed Central, in addition to its role as an archive, lies in the availability of data from diverse sources stored in a common format in a single repository. Many journals already have online publishing operations, and there is a growing tendency to publish material online only, to the exclusion of print.

[6] PubMed was developed by the National Center for Biotechnology Information (NCBI) at the National Library of Medicine (NLM) at the National Institutes of Health (NIH). The PubMed database was developed in conjunction with publishers of biomedical literature as a search tool for accessing literature citations and linking to full-text journal articles at Web sites of participating publishers. Publishers that participate in PubMed supply NLM with their citations electronically prior to or at the time of publication.

- **A double-blind comparative study of zolpidem versus zopiclone in the treatment of chronic primary insomnia.**
  Author(s): Tsutsui S; Zolipidem Study Group.
  Source: J Int Med Res. 2001 May-June; 29(3): 163-77.
  http://www.ncbi.nlm.nih.gov:80/entrez/query.fcgi?cmd=Retrieve&db=PubMed&list_uids=11471853&dopt=Abstract

- **A double-blind, randomized and placebo-controlled study on the polysomnographic withdrawal effects of zopiclone, zolpidem and triazolam in healthy subjects.**
  Author(s): Voderholzer U, Riemann D, Hornyak M, Backhaus J, Feige B, Berger M, Hohagen F.
  Source: European Archives of Psychiatry and Clinical Neuroscience. 2001 June; 251(3): 117-23.
  http://www.ncbi.nlm.nih.gov:80/entrez/query.fcgi?cmd=Retrieve&db=PubMed&list_uids=11697572&dopt=Abstract

- **Abuse, dependence, and epileptic seizures after zolpidem withdrawal: review and case report.**
  Author(s): Aragona M.
  Source: Clinical Neuropharmacology. 2000 September-October; 23(5): 281-3. Review.
  http://www.ncbi.nlm.nih.gov:80/entrez/query.fcgi?cmd=Retrieve&db=PubMed&list_uids=11154097&dopt=Abstract

- **Acute behavioral effects and abuse potential of trazodone, zolpidem and triazolam in humans.**
  Author(s): Rush CR, Baker RW, Wright K.
  Source: Psychopharmacology. 1999 June; 144(3): 220-33.
  http://www.ncbi.nlm.nih.gov:80/entrez/query.fcgi?cmd=Retrieve&db=PubMed&list_uids=10435388&dopt=Abstract

- **Acute zolpidem overdose leading to coma and respiratory failure.**
  Author(s): Hamad A, Sharma N.
  Source: Intensive Care Medicine. 2001 July; 27(7): 1239.
  http://www.ncbi.nlm.nih.gov:80/entrez/query.fcgi?cmd=Retrieve&db=PubMed&list_uids=11534578&dopt=Abstract

- **Acute zolpidem overdose--report of two cases.**
  Author(s): Gock SB, Wong SH, Nuwayhid N, Venuti SE, Kelley PD, Teggatz JR, Jentzen JM.
  Source: Journal of Analytical Toxicology. 1999 October; 23(6): 559-62.
  http://www.ncbi.nlm.nih.gov:80/entrez/query.fcgi?cmd=Retrieve&db=PubMed&list_uids=10517569&dopt=Abstract

- **Arousal from a semi-comatose state on zolpidem.**
  Author(s): Clauss RP, van der Merwe CE, Nel HW.
  Source: South African Medical Journal. Suid-Afrikaanse Tydskrif Vir Geneeskunde. 2001 October; 91(10): 788-9.
  http://www.ncbi.nlm.nih.gov:80/entrez/query.fcgi?cmd=Retrieve&db=PubMed&list_uids=11732448&dopt=Abstract

- **Behavioral pharmacology of zolpidem relative to benzodiazepines: a review.**
  Author(s): Rush CR.
  Source: Pharmacology, Biochemistry, and Behavior. 1998 November; 61(3): 253-69. Review.
  http://www.ncbi.nlm.nih.gov:80/entrez/query.fcgi?cmd=Retrieve&db=PubMed&list_uids=9768560&dopt=Abstract

- **Beneficial effect of zolpidem for dementia.**
  Author(s): Jarry C, Fontenas JP, Jonville-Bera AP, Autret-Leca E.
  Source: The Annals of Pharmacotherapy. 2002 November; 36(11): 1808.
  http://www.ncbi.nlm.nih.gov:80/entrez/query.fcgi?cmd=Retrieve&db=PubMed&list_uids=12398580&dopt=Abstract

- **Central nervous system side effects associated with zolpidem treatment.**
  Author(s): Toner LC, Tsambiras BM, Catalano G, Catalano MC, Cooper DS.
  Source: Clinical Neuropharmacology. 2000 January-February; 23(1): 54-8. Review.
  http://www.ncbi.nlm.nih.gov:80/entrez/query.fcgi?cmd=Retrieve&db=PubMed&list_uids=10682233&dopt=Abstract

- **Clinical syndrome associated with zolpidem ingestion in dogs: 33 cases (January 1998-July 2000).**
  Author(s): Richardson JA, Gwaltney-Brant SM, Albretsen JC, Khan SA, Porter JA.
  Source: J Vet Intern Med. 2002 March-April; 16(2): 208-10.
  http://www.ncbi.nlm.nih.gov:80/entrez/query.fcgi?cmd=Retrieve&db=PubMed&list_uids=11899040&dopt=Abstract

- **Clinically important drug interactions with zopiclone, zolpidem and zaleplon.**
  Author(s): Hesse LM, von Moltke LL, Greenblatt DJ.
  Source: Cns Drugs. 2003; 17(7): 513-32. Review.
  http://www.ncbi.nlm.nih.gov:80/entrez/query.fcgi?cmd=Retrieve&db=PubMed&list_uids=12751920&dopt=Abstract

- **Coadministration of short-term zolpidem with sertraline in healthy women.**
  Author(s): Allard S, Sainati SM, Roth-Schechter BF.
  Source: Journal of Clinical Pharmacology. 1999 February; 39(2): 184-91.
  http://www.ncbi.nlm.nih.gov:80/entrez/query.fcgi?cmd=Retrieve&db=PubMed&list_uids=11563412&dopt=Abstract

- **Comparative kinetics and dynamics of zaleplon, zolpidem, and placebo.**
  Author(s): Greenblatt DJ, Harmatz JS, von Moltke LL, Ehrenberg BL, Harrel L, Corbett K, Counihan M, Graf JA, Darwish M, Mertzanis P, Martin PT, Cevallos WH, Shader RI.
  Source: Clinical Pharmacology and Therapeutics. 1998 November; 64(5): 553-61.
  http://www.ncbi.nlm.nih.gov:80/entrez/query.fcgi?cmd=Retrieve&db=PubMed&list_uids=9834048&dopt=Abstract

- **Comparative kinetics and response to the benzodiazepine agonists triazolam and zolpidem: evaluation of sex-dependent differences.**
  Author(s): Greenblatt DJ, Harmatz JS, von Moltke LL, Wright CE, Durol AL, Harrel-Joseph LM, Shader RI.
  Source: The Journal of Pharmacology and Experimental Therapeutics. 2000 May; 293(2): 435-43.
  http://www.ncbi.nlm.nih.gov:80/entrez/query.fcgi?cmd=Retrieve&db=PubMed&list_uids=10773013&dopt=Abstract

- **Comparative tolerability, pharmacodynamics, and pharmacokinetics of a metabolite of a quinolizinone hypnotic and zolpidem in healthy subjects.**
  Author(s): Dingemanse J, Bury M, Hussain Y, van Giersbergen P.
  Source: Drug Metabolism and Disposition: the Biological Fate of Chemicals. 2000 December; 28(12): 1411-6.
  http://www.ncbi.nlm.nih.gov:80/entrez/query.fcgi?cmd=Retrieve&db=PubMed&list_uids=11095577&dopt=Abstract

- **Comparison of the effects of zaleplon, zolpidem, and triazolam at various GABA(A) receptor subtypes.**
  Author(s): Sanna E, Busonero F, Talani G, Carta M, Massa F, Peis M, Maciocco E, Biggio G.
  Source: European Journal of Pharmacology. 2002 September 13; 451(2): 103-10.
  http://www.ncbi.nlm.nih.gov:80/entrez/query.fcgi?cmd=Retrieve&db=PubMed&list_uids=12231378&dopt=Abstract

- **Comparison of the effects of zaleplon, zolpidem, and triazolam on memory, learning, and psychomotor performance.**
  Author(s): Troy SM, Lucki I, Unruh MA, Cevallos WH, Leister CA, Martin PT, Furlan PM, Mangano R.
  Source: Journal of Clinical Psychopharmacology. 2000 June; 20(3): 328-37.
  http://www.ncbi.nlm.nih.gov:80/entrez/query.fcgi?cmd=Retrieve&db=PubMed&list_uids=10831020&dopt=Abstract

- **Comparison of the effects of zolpidem and triazolam on nocturnal sleep and sleep latency in the morning: a cross-over study in healthy young volunteers.**
  Author(s): Kanno O, Sasaki T, Watanabe H, Takazawa S, Nakagome K, Nakajima T, Ichikawa I, Akaho R, Suzuki M.
  Source: Progress in Neuro-Psychopharmacology & Biological Psychiatry. 2000 August; 24(6): 897-910.
  http://www.ncbi.nlm.nih.gov:80/entrez/query.fcgi?cmd=Retrieve&db=PubMed&list_uids=11041533&dopt=Abstract

- **Comparison of the effects of zolpidem and zopiclone on nocturnal sleep and sleep latency in the morning: a cross-over study in healthy young volunteers.**
  Author(s): Nakajima T, Sasaki T, Nakagome K, Takazawa S, Ikebuchi E, Ito Y, Miyazawa Y, Tanaka M, Kanno O.
  Source: Life Sciences. 2000 May 26; 67(1): 81-90.
  http://www.ncbi.nlm.nih.gov:80/entrez/query.fcgi?cmd=Retrieve&db=PubMed&list_uids=10896032&dopt=Abstract

- **Continuous flumazenil infusion in the treatment of zolpidem (Ambien) and ethanol coingestion.**
  Author(s): Burton JH, Lyon L, Dorfman T, Tomassoni AJ.
  Source: Journal of Toxicology. Clinical Toxicology. 1998; 36(7): 743-6.
  http://www.ncbi.nlm.nih.gov:80/entrez/query.fcgi?cmd=Retrieve&db=PubMed&list_uids=9865246&dopt=Abstract

- **Continuous versus non-nightly use of zolpidem in chronic insomnia: results of a large-scale, double-blind, randomized, outpatient study.**
  Author(s): Hajak G, Cluydts R, Declerck A, Estivill SE, Middleton A, Sonka K, Unden M.
  Source: International Clinical Psychopharmacology. 2002 January; 17(1): 9-17. Erratum In: Int Clin Psychopharmacol 2002 July; 17(4): 206.
  http://www.ncbi.nlm.nih.gov:80/entrez/query.fcgi?cmd=Retrieve&db=PubMed&list_uids=11800507&dopt=Abstract

- **Conventional and power spectrum analysis of the effects of zolpidem on sleep EEG in patients with chronic primary insomnia.**
  Author(s): Monti JM, Alvarino F, Monti D.
  Source: Sleep. 2000 December 15; 23(8): 1075-84.
  http://www.ncbi.nlm.nih.gov:80/entrez/query.fcgi?cmd=Retrieve&db=PubMed&list_uids=11145322&dopt=Abstract

- **Delirium associated with zolpidem.**
  Author(s): Brodeur MR, Stirling AL.
  Source: The Annals of Pharmacotherapy. 2001 December; 35(12): 1562-4.
  http://www.ncbi.nlm.nih.gov:80/entrez/query.fcgi?cmd=Retrieve&db=PubMed&list_uids=11793620&dopt=Abstract

- **Dependence on zolpidem in high dose.**
  Author(s): Vartzopoulos D, Bozikas V, Phocas C, Karavatos A, Kaprinis G.
  Source: International Clinical Psychopharmacology. 2000 May; 15(3): 181-2.
  http://www.ncbi.nlm.nih.gov:80/entrez/query.fcgi?cmd=Retrieve&db=PubMed&list_uids=10870877&dopt=Abstract

- **Dependence on zolpidem: a case report.**
  Author(s): Sakkas P, Psarros C, Masdrakis V, Liappas J, Christodoulou GN.
  Source: European Psychiatry : the Journal of the Association of European Psychiatrists. 1999 October; 14(6): 358-9.
  http://www.ncbi.nlm.nih.gov:80/entrez/query.fcgi?cmd=Retrieve&db=PubMed&list_uids=10572372&dopt=Abstract

- **Differential effects in humans after repeated administrations of zolpidem and triazolam.**
  Author(s): Stoops WW, Rush CR.
  Source: The American Journal of Drug and Alcohol Abuse. 2003 May; 29(2): 281-99.
  http://www.ncbi.nlm.nih.gov:80/entrez/query.fcgi?cmd=Retrieve&db=PubMed&list_uids=12765207&dopt=Abstract

- **Differential impairment of triazolam and zolpidem clearance by ritonavir.**
  Author(s): Greenblatt DJ, von Moltke LL, Harmatz JS, Durol AL, Daily JP, Graf JA, Mertzanis P, Hoffman JL, Shader RI.
  Source: Journal of Acquired Immune Deficiency Syndromes (1999). 2000 June 1; 24(2): 129-36.
  http://www.ncbi.nlm.nih.gov:80/entrez/query.fcgi?cmd=Retrieve&db=PubMed&list_uids=10935688&dopt=Abstract

- **Discriminative-stimulus effects of zolpidem, triazolam, pentobarbital, and caffeine in zolpidem-trained humans.**
  Author(s): Rush CR, Baker RW, Rowlett JK.
  Source: Experimental and Clinical Psychopharmacology. 2000 February; 8(1): 22-36.
  http://www.ncbi.nlm.nih.gov:80/entrez/query.fcgi?cmd=Retrieve&db=PubMed&list_uids=10743902&dopt=Abstract

- **Effect of itraconazole on the pharmacokinetics and pharmacodynamics of zolpidem.**
  Author(s): Luurila H, Kivisto KT, Neuvonen PJ.
  Source: European Journal of Clinical Pharmacology. 1998 April; 54(2): 163-6.
  http://www.ncbi.nlm.nih.gov:80/entrez/query.fcgi?cmd=Retrieve&db=PubMed&list_uids=9626922&dopt=Abstract

- **Effect of zolpidem on human cytochrome P450 activity, and on transport mediated by P-glycoprotein.**
  Author(s): von Moltke LL, Weemhoff JL, Perloff MD, Hesse LM, Harmatz JS, Roth-Schechter BF, Greenblatt DJ.
  Source: Biopharmaceutics & Drug Disposition. 2002 December; 23(9): 361-7.
  http://www.ncbi.nlm.nih.gov:80/entrez/query.fcgi?cmd=Retrieve&db=PubMed&list_uids=12469329&dopt=Abstract

- **Effectiveness and tolerability of melatonin and zolpidem for the alleviation of jet lag.**
  Author(s): Suhner A, Schlagenhauf P, Hofer I, Johnson R, Tschopp A, Steffen R.
  Source: Aviation, Space, and Environmental Medicine. 2001 July; 72(7): 638-46.
  http://www.ncbi.nlm.nih.gov:80/entrez/query.fcgi?cmd=Retrieve&db=PubMed&list_uids=11471907&dopt=Abstract

- **Effects of alcohol, zolpidem, and some other sedatives and hypnotics on human performance and memory.**
  Author(s): Mattila MJ, Vanakoski J, Kalska H, Seppala T.
  Source: Pharmacology, Biochemistry, and Behavior. 1998 April; 59(4): 917-23.
  http://www.ncbi.nlm.nih.gov:80/entrez/query.fcgi?cmd=Retrieve&db=PubMed&list_uids=9586849&dopt=Abstract

- **Effects of alprazolam, caffeine, and zolpidem in humans trained to discriminate triazolam from placebo.**
  Author(s): Smith BJ, Bickel WK.
  Source: Drug and Alcohol Dependence. 2001 February 1; 61(3): 249-60.
  http://www.ncbi.nlm.nih.gov:80/entrez/query.fcgi?cmd=Retrieve&db=PubMed&list_uids=11164689&dopt=Abstract

- **Effects of zolpidem 10 mg, zopiclone 7.5 mg and flunitrazepam 1 mg on night-time motor activity.**
  Author(s): Denise P, Bocca ML.
  Source: European Neuropsychopharmacology : the Journal of the European College of Neuropsychopharmacology. 2003 March; 13(2): 111-5.
  http://www.ncbi.nlm.nih.gov:80/entrez/query.fcgi?cmd=Retrieve&db=PubMed&list_uids=12650955&dopt=Abstract

- **Eight weeks of non-nightly use of zolpidem for primary insomnia.**
  Author(s): Walsh JK, Roth T, Randazzo A, Erman M, Jamieson A, Scharf M, Schweitzer PK, Ware JC.
  Source: Sleep. 2000 December 15; 23(8): 1087-96.
  http://www.ncbi.nlm.nih.gov:80/entrez/query.fcgi?cmd=Retrieve&db=PubMed&list_uids=11145323&dopt=Abstract

- **Epidemiological evidence for a low abuse potential of zolpidem.**
  Author(s): Soyka M, Bottlender R, Moller HJ.
  Source: Pharmacopsychiatry. 2000 July; 33(4): 138-41. Review.
  http://www.ncbi.nlm.nih.gov:80/entrez/query.fcgi?cmd=Retrieve&db=PubMed&list_uids=10958262&dopt=Abstract

- **GC/MS determination of zolpidem in postmortem specimens in a voluntary intoxication.**
  Author(s): Keller T, Schneider A, Tutsch-Bauer E.
  Source: Forensic Science International. 1999 December 6; 106(2): 103-8.
  http://www.ncbi.nlm.nih.gov:80/entrez/query.fcgi?cmd=Retrieve&db=PubMed&list_uids=10664896&dopt=Abstract

- **Hepatotoxicity associated with zolpidem treatment.**
  Author(s): Karsenti D, Blanc P, Bacq Y, Metman EH.
  Source: Bmj (Clinical Research Ed.). 1999 May 1; 318(7192): 1179.
  http://www.ncbi.nlm.nih.gov:80/entrez/query.fcgi?cmd=Retrieve&db=PubMed&list_uids=10221943&dopt=Abstract

- **Ineffectiveness of intermittent zolpidem.**
  Author(s): Kripke DF.
  Source: Sleep Medicine Reviews. 2003 April; 7(2): 193; Author Reply 195-6.
  http://www.ncbi.nlm.nih.gov:80/entrez/query.fcgi?cmd=Retrieve&db=PubMed&list_uids=12628218&dopt=Abstract

- **Kinetic and dynamic interaction study of zolpidem with ketoconazole, itraconazole, and fluconazole.**
  Author(s): Greenblatt DJ, von Moltke LL, Harmatz JS, Mertzanis P, Graf JA, Durol AL, Counihan M, Roth-Schechter B, Shader RI.
  Source: Clinical Pharmacology and Therapeutics. 1998 December; 64(6): 661-71.
  http://www.ncbi.nlm.nih.gov:80/entrez/query.fcgi?cmd=Retrieve&db=PubMed&list_uids=9871431&dopt=Abstract

- **Lack of cross-reactivity of Ambien (zolpidem) with drugs in standard urine drug screens.**
  Author(s): Piergies AA, Sainati S, Roth-Schechter B.
  Source: Archives of Pathology & Laboratory Medicine. 1997 April; 121(4): 392-4.
  http://www.ncbi.nlm.nih.gov:80/entrez/query.fcgi?cmd=Retrieve&db=PubMed&list_uids=9140309&dopt=Abstract

- **Metabolism of anxiolytics and hypnotics: benzodiazepines, buspirone, zoplicone, and zolpidem.**
  Author(s): Chouinard G, Lefko-Singh K, Teboul E.
  Source: Cellular and Molecular Neurobiology. 1999 August; 19(4): 533-52. Review.
  http://www.ncbi.nlm.nih.gov:80/entrez/query.fcgi?cmd=Retrieve&db=PubMed&list_uids=10379424&dopt=Abstract

- **Minimal interaction between fluoxetine and multiple-dose zolpidem in healthy women.**
  Author(s): Allard S, Sainati S, Roth-Schechter B, MacIntyre J.
  Source: Drug Metabolism and Disposition: the Biological Fate of Chemicals. 1998 July; 26(7): 617-22.
  http://www.ncbi.nlm.nih.gov:80/entrez/query.fcgi?cmd=Retrieve&db=PubMed&list_uids=9660843&dopt=Abstract

- **New drugs for insomnia: comparative tolerability of zopiclone, zolpidem and zaleplon.**
  Author(s): Terzano MG, Rossi M, Palomba V, Smerieri A, Parrino L.
  Source: Drug Safety : an International Journal of Medical Toxicology and Drug Experience. 2003; 26(4): 261-82. Review.
  http://www.ncbi.nlm.nih.gov:80/entrez/query.fcgi?cmd=Retrieve&db=PubMed&list_uids=12608888&dopt=Abstract

- **Pharmacokinetics, pharmacodynamics, and relative pharmacokinetic/pharmacodynamic profiles of zaleplon and zolpidem.**
  Author(s): Drover D, Lemmens H, Naidu S, Cevallos W, Darwish M, Stanski D.
  Source: Clinical Therapeutics. 2000 December; 22(12): 1443-61.
  http://www.ncbi.nlm.nih.gov:80/entrez/query.fcgi?cmd=Retrieve&db=PubMed&list_uids=11192136&dopt=Abstract

- **Placebo-controlled sleep laboratory studies on the acute effects of zolpidem on objective and subjective sleep and awakening quality in nonorganic insomnia related to neurotic and stress-related disorder.**
  Author(s): Saletu-Zyhlarz G, Anderer P, Brandstatter N, Dantendorfer K, Gruber G, Mandl M, Ritter K, Zoghlami A, Saletu B.
  Source: Neuropsychobiology. 2000; 41(3): 139-48.
  http://www.ncbi.nlm.nih.gov:80/entrez/query.fcgi?cmd=Retrieve&db=PubMed&list_uids=10754428&dopt=Abstract

- **Polysomnographic findings during non-continuous administration of zolpidem.**
  Author(s): Cluydts R, Heyde K, De Volder I.
  Source: Sleep Medicine Reviews. 2002 October; 6 Suppl 1: S13-9; Discussion S19.
  http://www.ncbi.nlm.nih.gov:80/entrez/query.fcgi?cmd=Retrieve&db=PubMed&list_uids=12607572&dopt=Abstract

- **Residual effect of zolpidem 10 mg and zopiclone 7.5 mg versus flunitrazepam 1 mg and placebo on driving performance and ocular saccades.**
  Author(s): Bocca ML, Le Doze F, Etard O, Pottier M, L'Hoste J, Denise P.
  Source: Psychopharmacology. 1999 April; 143(4): 373-9.
  http://www.ncbi.nlm.nih.gov:80/entrez/query.fcgi?cmd=Retrieve&db=PubMed&list_uids=10367554&dopt=Abstract

- **Residual effects of middle-of-the-night administration of zaleplon and zolpidem on driving ability, memory functions, and psychomotor performance.**
  Author(s): Verster JC, Volkerts ER, Schreuder AH, Eijken EJ, van Heuckelum JH, Veldhuijzen DS, Verbaten MN, Paty I, Darwish M, Danjou P, Patat A.
  Source: Journal of Clinical Psychopharmacology. 2002 December; 22(6): 576-83.
  http://www.ncbi.nlm.nih.gov:80/entrez/query.fcgi?cmd=Retrieve&db=PubMed&list_uids=12454557&dopt=Abstract

- **Safety and tolerance of zolpidem in the treatment of disturbed sleep: a post-marketing surveillance of 16944 cases.**
  Author(s): Hajak G, Bandelow B.
  Source: International Clinical Psychopharmacology. 1998 July; 13(4): 157-67.
  http://www.ncbi.nlm.nih.gov:80/entrez/query.fcgi?cmd=Retrieve&db=PubMed&list_uids=9727726&dopt=Abstract

- **Seizures associated with venlafaxine, methylphenidate, and zolpidem.**
  Author(s): Tavakoli SA, Gleason OC.
  Source: Psychosomatics. 2003 May-June; 44(3): 262-4.
  http://www.ncbi.nlm.nih.gov:80/entrez/query.fcgi?cmd=Retrieve&db=PubMed&list_uids=12724513&dopt=Abstract

- **Selective effects of zolpidem on human memory functions.**
  Author(s): Mintzer MZ, Griffiths RR.
  Source: Journal of Psychopharmacology (Oxford, England). 1999; 13(1): 18-31.
  http://www.ncbi.nlm.nih.gov:80/entrez/query.fcgi?cmd=Retrieve&db=PubMed&list_uids=10221356&dopt=Abstract

- **Soyka M, Bottlender R, Moller H-J; Epidemiological evidence for a low abuse potential of zolpidem; Pharmacopsychiatry 2000, 33: 138-141.**
  Author(s): Engfer A.
  Source: Pharmacopsychiatry. 2002 March; 35(2): 81; Author Reply 81-2.
  http://www.ncbi.nlm.nih.gov:80/entrez/query.fcgi?cmd=Retrieve&db=PubMed&list_uids=11951152&dopt=Abstract

- **Species differences in regional patterns of 3H-8-OH-DPAT and 3H-zolpidem binding in the rat and human brain.**
  Author(s): Duncan GE, Knapp DJ, Breese GR, Crews FT, Little KY.
  Source: Pharmacology, Biochemistry, and Behavior. 1998 June; 60(2): 439-48.
  http://www.ncbi.nlm.nih.gov:80/entrez/query.fcgi?cmd=Retrieve&db=PubMed&list_uids=9632227&dopt=Abstract

- **Subhypnotic doses of zolpidem oppose dopaminergic-induced dyskinesia in Parkinson's disease.**
  Author(s): Ruzicka E, Roth J, Jech R, Busek P.
  Source: Movement Disorders : Official Journal of the Movement Disorder Society. 2000 July; 15(4): 734-5.
  http://www.ncbi.nlm.nih.gov:80/entrez/query.fcgi?cmd=Retrieve&db=PubMed&list_uids=10928588&dopt=Abstract

- **Temazepam, but not zolpidem, causes orthostatic hypotension in astronauts after spaceflight.**
  Author(s): Shi SJ, Garcia KM, Meck JV.
  Source: Journal of Cardiovascular Pharmacology. 2003 January; 41(1): 31-9.
  http://www.ncbi.nlm.nih.gov:80/entrez/query.fcgi?cmd=Retrieve&db=PubMed&list_uids=12500019&dopt=Abstract

- **Temperature-dependent effect of zolpidem on the GABAA receptor-mediated response at recombinant human GABAA receptor subtypes.**
  Author(s): Munakata M, Jin YH, Akaike N, Nielsen M.
  Source: Brain Research. 1998 October 5; 807(1-2): 199-202.
  http://www.ncbi.nlm.nih.gov:80/entrez/query.fcgi?cmd=Retrieve&db=PubMed&list_uids=9757036&dopt=Abstract

- **The abuse potential of zolpidem administered alone and with alcohol.**
  Author(s): Wilkinson CJ.
  Source: Pharmacology, Biochemistry, and Behavior. 1998 May; 60(1): 193-202.
  http://www.ncbi.nlm.nih.gov:80/entrez/query.fcgi?cmd=Retrieve&db=PubMed&list_uids=9610942&dopt=Abstract

- **The effect of zolpidem and zopiclone on memory.**
  Author(s): Isawa S, Suzuki M, Uchiumi M, Murasaki M.
  Source: Nihon Shinkei Seishin Yakurigaku Zasshi. 2000 May; 20(2): 61-9.
  http://www.ncbi.nlm.nih.gov:80/entrez/query.fcgi?cmd=Retrieve&db=PubMed&list_uids=11062863&dopt=Abstract

- **The effects of zolpidem and zopiclone on daytime sleepiness and psychomotor performance.**
  Author(s): Uchiumi M, Isawa S, Suzuki M, Murasaki M.
  Source: Nihon Shinkei Seishin Yakurigaku Zasshi. 2000 August; 20(3): 123-30.
  http://www.ncbi.nlm.nih.gov:80/entrez/query.fcgi?cmd=Retrieve&db=PubMed&list_uids=11215153&dopt=Abstract

- **The safety and tolerability of zolpidem—an update.**
  Author(s): Darcourt G, Pringuey D, Salliere D, Lavoisy J.
  Source: Journal of Psychopharmacology (Oxford, England). 1999; 13(1): 81-93. Review.
  http://www.ncbi.nlm.nih.gov:80/entrez/query.fcgi?cmd=Retrieve&db=PubMed&list_uids=10221362&dopt=Abstract

- **Three cases of zolpidem dependence treated with fluoxetine: the serotonin hypothesis.**
  Author(s): Liappas IA, Malitas PN, Dimopoulos NP, Gitsa OE, Liappas AI, Nikolaou CK, Christodoulou GN.
  Source: World J Biol Psychiatry. 2003 April; 4(2): 93-6.
  http://www.ncbi.nlm.nih.gov:80/entrez/query.fcgi?cmd=Retrieve&db=PubMed&list_uids=12692780&dopt=Abstract

- **Triazolam and zolpidem: a comparison of their psychomotor, cognitive, and subjective effects in healthy volunteers.**
  Author(s): Mintzer MZ, Frey JM, Yingling JE, Griffiths RR.
  Source: Behavioural Pharmacology. 1997 November; 8(6-7): 561-74.
  http://www.ncbi.nlm.nih.gov:80/entrez/query.fcgi?cmd=Retrieve&db=PubMed&list_uids=9832970&dopt=Abstract

- **Triazolam and zolpidem: effects on human memory and attentional processes.**
  Author(s): Mintzer MZ, Griffiths RR.
  Source: Psychopharmacology. 1999 May; 144(1): 8-19.
  http://www.ncbi.nlm.nih.gov:80/entrez/query.fcgi?cmd=Retrieve&db=PubMed&list_uids=10379619&dopt=Abstract

- **Validation of a method for the determination of zolpidem in human plasma using LC with fluorescence detection.**
  Author(s): Ring PR, Bostick JM.
  Source: Journal of Pharmaceutical and Biomedical Analysis. 2000 April; 22(3): 495-504.
  http://www.ncbi.nlm.nih.gov:80/entrez/query.fcgi?cmd=Retrieve&db=PubMed&list_uids=10766367&dopt=Abstract

- **Zolpidem "as needed" for the treatment of primary insomnia: a double-blind, placebo-controlled study.**
  Author(s): Walsh JK.
  Source: Sleep Medicine Reviews. 2002 October; 6 Suppl 1: S7-10; Discussion S10-1, S31-3.
  http://www.ncbi.nlm.nih.gov:80/entrez/query.fcgi?cmd=Retrieve&db=PubMed&list_uids=12607571&dopt=Abstract

- **Zolpidem "as needed" versus continuous administration: Pan-European study results.**
  Author(s): Hajak G.
  Source: Sleep Medicine Reviews. 2002 October; 6 Suppl 1: S21-8; Discussion S31-3.
  http://www.ncbi.nlm.nih.gov:80/entrez/query.fcgi?cmd=Retrieve&db=PubMed&list_uids=12607573&dopt=Abstract

- **Zolpidem (Ambien): a pediatric case series.**
  Author(s): Kurta DL, Myers LB, Krenzelok EP.
  Source: Journal of Toxicology. Clinical Toxicology. 1997; 35(5): 453-7.
  http://www.ncbi.nlm.nih.gov:80/entrez/query.fcgi?cmd=Retrieve&db=PubMed&list_uids=9279301&dopt=Abstract

- **Zolpidem 10 mg given at daytime is not antagonized by 300 mg caffeine in man.**
  Author(s): Mattila MJ, Nurminen ML, Vainio P, Vanakoski J.
  Source: European Journal of Clinical Pharmacology. 1998 July; 54(5): 421-5.
  http://www.ncbi.nlm.nih.gov:80/entrez/query.fcgi?cmd=Retrieve&db=PubMed&list_uids=9754987&dopt=Abstract

- **Zolpidem abuse.**
  Author(s): Madrak LN, Rosenberg M.
  Source: The American Journal of Psychiatry. 2001 August; 158(8): 1330-1.
  http://www.ncbi.nlm.nih.gov:80/entrez/query.fcgi?cmd=Retrieve&db=PubMed&list_uids=11481176&dopt=Abstract

- **Zolpidem and driving impairment.**
  Author(s): Logan BK, Couper FJ.
  Source: J Forensic Sci. 2001 January; 46(1): 105-10.
  http://www.ncbi.nlm.nih.gov:80/entrez/query.fcgi?cmd=Retrieve&db=PubMed&list_uids=11210892&dopt=Abstract

- **Zolpidem and promethazine in pre-anaesthetic medication. A pharmacopsychological approach.**
  Author(s): Uhlig T, Huppe M, Brand K, Heinze J, Schmucker P.
  Source: Neuropsychobiology. 2000; 42(3): 139-48.
  http://www.ncbi.nlm.nih.gov:80/entrez/query.fcgi?cmd=Retrieve&db=PubMed&list_uids=11015032&dopt=Abstract

- **Zolpidem dependence and prescription fraud.**
  Author(s): Golden SA, Vagnoni C.
  Source: The American Journal on Addictions / American Academy of Psychiatrists in Alcoholism and Addictions. 2000 Winter; 9(1): 96-7.
  http://www.ncbi.nlm.nih.gov:80/entrez/query.fcgi?cmd=Retrieve&db=PubMed&list_uids=10914300&dopt=Abstract

- **Zolpidem dependence case series: possible neurobiological mechanisms and clinical management.**
  Author(s): Liappas IA, Malitas PN, Dimopoulos NP, Gitsa OE, Liappas AI, Nikolaou ChK, Christodoulou GN.
  Source: Journal of Psychopharmacology (Oxford, England). 2003 March; 17(1): 131-5.
  http://www.ncbi.nlm.nih.gov:80/entrez/query.fcgi?cmd=Retrieve&db=PubMed&list_uids=12680751&dopt=Abstract

- **Zolpidem distribution in postmortem cases.**
  Author(s): Levine B, Wu SC, Smialek JE.
  Source: J Forensic Sci. 1999 March; 44(2): 369-71.
  http://www.ncbi.nlm.nih.gov:80/entrez/query.fcgi?cmd=Retrieve&db=PubMed&list_uids=10097364&dopt=Abstract

- **Zolpidem for antipsychotic-induced parkinsonism.**
  Author(s): Farver DK, Khan MH.
  Source: The Annals of Pharmacotherapy. 2001 April; 35(4): 435-7.
  http://www.ncbi.nlm.nih.gov:80/entrez/query.fcgi?cmd=Retrieve&db=PubMed&list_uids=11302407&dopt=Abstract

- **Zolpidem for insomnia related to PTSD.**
  Author(s): Dieperink ME, Drogemuller L.
  Source: Psychiatric Services (Washington, D.C.). 1999 March; 50(3): 421.
  http://www.ncbi.nlm.nih.gov:80/entrez/query.fcgi?cmd=Retrieve&db=PubMed&list_uids=10096658&dopt=Abstract

- **Zolpidem for persistent insomnia in SSRI-treated depressed patients.**
  Author(s): Asnis GM, Chakraburtty A, DuBoff EA, Krystal A, Londborg PD, Rosenberg R, Roth-Schechter B, Scharf MB, Walsh JK.
  Source: The Journal of Clinical Psychiatry. 1999 October; 60(10): 668-76.
  http://www.ncbi.nlm.nih.gov:80/entrez/query.fcgi?cmd=Retrieve&db=PubMed&list_uids=10549683&dopt=Abstract

- **Zolpidem improves dystonia in "Lubag" or X-linked dystonia-parkinsonism syndrome.**
  Author(s): Evidente VG.
  Source: Neurology. 2002 February 26; 58(4): 662-3.
  http://www.ncbi.nlm.nih.gov:80/entrez/query.fcgi?cmd=Retrieve&db=PubMed&list_uids=11865155&dopt=Abstract

- **Zolpidem in progressive supranuclear palsy.**
  Author(s): Daniele A, Moro E, Bentivoglio AR.
  Source: The New England Journal of Medicine. 1999 August 12; 341(7): 543-4. Erratum In: N Engl J Med 1999 November 18; 341(21): 1632.
  http://www.ncbi.nlm.nih.gov:80/entrez/query.fcgi?cmd=Retrieve&db=PubMed&list_uids=10447452&dopt=Abstract

- **Zolpidem in progressive supranuclear palsy.**
  Author(s): Mayr BJ, Bonelli RM, Niederwieser G, Koltringer P, Reisecker F.
  Source: European Journal of Neurology : the Official Journal of the European Federation of Neurological Societies. 2002 March; 9(2): 184-5.
  http://www.ncbi.nlm.nih.gov:80/entrez/query.fcgi?cmd=Retrieve&db=PubMed&list_uids=11882066&dopt=Abstract

- **Zolpidem in restless legs syndrome.**
  Author(s): Bezerra ML, Martinez JV.
  Source: European Neurology. 2002; 48(3): 180-1.
  http://www.ncbi.nlm.nih.gov:80/entrez/query.fcgi?cmd=Retrieve&db=PubMed&list_uids=12373037&dopt=Abstract

- **Zolpidem is differentiated from triazolam in humans using a three-response drug discrimination procedure.**
  Author(s): Mintzer MZ, Frey JM, Griffiths RR.
  Source: Behavioural Pharmacology. 1998 November; 9(7): 545-59.
  http://www.ncbi.nlm.nih.gov:80/entrez/query.fcgi?cmd=Retrieve&db=PubMed&list_uids=9862080&dopt=Abstract

- **Zolpidem metabolism in vitro: responsible cytochromes, chemical inhibitors, and in vivo correlations.**
  Author(s): Von Moltke LL, Greenblatt DJ, Granda BW, Duan SX, Grassi JM, Venkatakrishnan K, Harmatz JS, Shader RI.
  Source: British Journal of Clinical Pharmacology. 1999 July; 48(1): 89-97.
  http://www.ncbi.nlm.nih.gov:80/entrez/query.fcgi?cmd=Retrieve&db=PubMed&list_uids=10383565&dopt=Abstract

- **Zolpidem pharmacokinetic properties in young females: influence of smoking and oral contraceptive use.**
  Author(s): Olubodun JO, Ochs HR, Truten V, Klein A, von Moltke LL, Harmatz JS, Shader RI, Greenblatt DJ.
  Source: Journal of Clinical Pharmacology. 2002 October; 42(10): 1142-6.
  http://www.ncbi.nlm.nih.gov:80/entrez/query.fcgi?cmd=Retrieve&db=PubMed&list_uids=12362929&dopt=Abstract

- **Zolpidem tartrate and somnambulism.**
  Author(s): Harazin J, Berigan TR.
  Source: Military Medicine. 1999 September; 164(9): 669-70.
  http://www.ncbi.nlm.nih.gov:80/entrez/query.fcgi?cmd=Retrieve&db=PubMed&list_uids=10495642&dopt=Abstract

- **Zolpidem tissue concentrations in a multiple drug related death involving Ambien.**
  Author(s): Meeker JE, Som CW, Macapagal EC, Benson PA.
  Source: Journal of Analytical Toxicology. 1995 October; 19(6): 531-4.
  http://www.ncbi.nlm.nih.gov:80/entrez/query.fcgi?cmd=Retrieve&db=PubMed&list_uids=8926752&dopt=Abstract

- **Zolpidem use and hip fractures in older people.**
  Author(s): Wang PS, Bohn RL, Glynn RJ, Mogun H, Avorn J.
  Source: Journal of the American Geriatrics Society. 2001 December; 49(12): 1685-90.
  http://www.ncbi.nlm.nih.gov:80/entrez/query.fcgi?cmd=Retrieve&db=PubMed&list_uids=11844004&dopt=Abstract

- **Zolpidem, a valuable alternative to benzodiazepine hypnotics for chronic insomnia?**
  Author(s): Declerck A, Smits M.
  Source: J Int Med Res. 1999; 27(6): 253-63. Erratum In: J Int Med Res 2000; 28(1): 46.
  http://www.ncbi.nlm.nih.gov:80/entrez/query.fcgi?cmd=Retrieve&db=PubMed&list_uids=10726234&dopt=Abstract

- **Zolpidem, vascular headache, and hallucinations in an adolescent.**
  Author(s): Andrade C.
  Source: The Australian and New Zealand Journal of Psychiatry. 2002 June; 36(3): 425-6.
  http://www.ncbi.nlm.nih.gov:80/entrez/query.fcgi?cmd=Retrieve&db=PubMed&list_uids=12060196&dopt=Abstract

- **Zolpidem: an update of its pharmacology, therapeutic efficacy and tolerability in the treatment of insomnia.**
  Author(s): Holm KJ, Goa KL.
  Source: Drugs. 2000 April; 59(4): 865-89. Review.
  http://www.ncbi.nlm.nih.gov:80/entrez/query.fcgi?cmd=Retrieve&db=PubMed&list_uids=10804040&dopt=Abstract

- **Zolpidem-associated hallucinations and serotonin reuptake inhibition: a possible interaction.**
  Author(s): Elko CJ, Burgess JL, Robertson WO.
  Source: Journal of Toxicology. Clinical Toxicology. 1998; 36(3): 195-203. Review.
  http://www.ncbi.nlm.nih.gov:80/entrez/query.fcgi?cmd=Retrieve&db=PubMed&list_uids=9656974&dopt=Abstract

- **Zolpidem-induced distortion in visual perception.**
  Author(s): Huang CL, Chang CJ, Hung CF, Lin HY.
  Source: The Annals of Pharmacotherapy. 2003 May; 37(5): 683-6. Review.
  http://www.ncbi.nlm.nih.gov:80/entrez/query.fcgi?cmd=Retrieve&db=PubMed&list_uids=12708947&dopt=Abstract

- **Zolpidem-related delirium: a case report.**
  Author(s): Freudenreich O, Menza M.
  Source: The Journal of Clinical Psychiatry. 2000 June; 61(6): 449-50.
  http://www.ncbi.nlm.nih.gov:80/entrez/query.fcgi?cmd=Retrieve&db=PubMed&list_uids=10901348&dopt=Abstract

- **Zolpidem-related epileptic seizures: a case report.**
  Author(s): Tripodianakis J, Potagas C, Papageorgiou P, Lazaridou M, Matikas N.
  Source: European Psychiatry : the Journal of the Association of European Psychiatrists. 2003 May; 18(3): 140-1.
  http://www.ncbi.nlm.nih.gov:80/entrez/query.fcgi?cmd=Retrieve&db=PubMed&list_uids=12763302&dopt=Abstract

CHAPTER 2. NUTRITION AND AMBIEN

Overview

In this chapter, we will show you how to find studies dedicated specifically to nutrition and Ambien.

Finding Nutrition Studies on Ambien

The National Institutes of Health's Office of Dietary Supplements (ODS) offers a searchable bibliographic database called the IBIDS (International Bibliographic Information on Dietary Supplements; National Institutes of Health, Building 31, Room 1B29, 31 Center Drive, MSC 2086, Bethesda, Maryland 20892-2086, Tel: 301-435-2920, Fax: 301-480-1845, E-mail: ods@nih.gov). The IBIDS contains over 460,000 scientific citations and summaries about dietary supplements and nutrition as well as references to published international, scientific literature on dietary supplements such as vitamins, minerals, and botanicals.[7] The IBIDS includes references and citations to both human and animal research studies.

As a service of the ODS, access to the IBIDS database is available free of charge at the following Web address: **http://ods.od.nih.gov/databases/ibids.html** After entering the search area, you have three choices: (1) IBIDS Consumer Database, (2) Full IBIDS Database, or (3) Peer Reviewed Citations Only.

Now that you have selected a database, click on the "Advanced" tab. An advanced search allows you to retrieve up to 100 fully explained references in a comprehensive format. Type "Ambien" (or synonyms) into the search box, and click "Go." To narrow the search, you can also select the "Title" field.

---

[7] Adapted from **http://ods.od.nih.gov**. IBIDS is produced by the Office of Dietary Supplements (ODS) at the National Institutes of Health to assist the public, healthcare providers, educators, and researchers in locating credible, scientific information on dietary supplements. IBIDS was developed and will be maintained through an interagency partnership with the Food and Nutrition Information Center of the National Agricultural Library, U.S. Department of Agriculture.

The following information is typical of that found when using the "Full IBIDS Database" to search for "Ambien" (or a synonym):

- **Cerebral blood perfusion after treatment with zolpidem and flumazenil in the baboon.**
  Author(s): Nuclear Medicine Department, Medical University of Southern Africa, Medunsa, South Africa.
  Source: Clauss, R P Dormehl, I C Kilian, E Louw, W K Nel, W H Oliver, D W Arzneimittelforschung. 2002; 52(10): 740-4 0004-4172

- **Clinical syndrome associated with zolpidem ingestion in dogs: 33 cases (January 1998-July 2000).**
  Author(s): ASPCA Animal Poison Control Center, Urbana, IL, USA. jar@napcc.aspca.org
  Source: Richardson, J A Gwaltney Brant, S M Albretsen, J C Khan, S A Porter, J A J-Vet-Intern-Med. 2002 Mar-April; 16(2): 208-10 0891-6640

- **Complexation of zolpidem with 2-hydroxypropyl-beta-, methyl-beta-, and 2-hydroxypropyl-gamma-cyclodextrin: effect on aqueous solubility, dissolution rate, and ataxic activity in rat.**
  Author(s): Dipartimento Farmaco-Chimico, Facolta di Farmacia, Universita degli Studi di Bari, Via Orabona 4, 70125 Bari, Italy. trapani@farmchim.uniba.it
  Source: Trapani, G Latrofa, A Franco, M Pantaleo, M R Sanna, E Massa, F Tuveri, F Liso, G J-Pharm-Sci. 2000 November; 89(11): 1443-51 0022-3549

- **Continuous versus non-nightly use of zolpidem in chronic insomnia: results of a large-scale, double-blind, randomized, outpatient study.**
  Author(s): Department of Psychiatry and Psychotherapy, University of Regensburg, Germany. goeran.hajak@bkr-regensburg.de
  Source: Hajak, G Cluydts, R Declerck, A Estivill, S Eduard Middleton, A Sonka, K Unden, M Int-Clin-Psychopharmacol. 2002 January; 17(1): 9-17 0268-1315

- **Discriminative stimulus effects of zolpidem in pentobarbital-trained subjects: II. Comparison with triazolam and caffeine in humans.**
  Author(s): Department of Psychiatry and Human Behavior, University of Mississippi Medical Center, Jackson, USA.
  Source: Rush, C R Madakasira, S Goldman, N H Woolverton, W L Rowlett, J K J-Pharmacol-Exp-Ther. 1997 January; 280(1): 174-88 0022-3565

- **Discriminative-stimulus effects of zolpidem, triazolam, pentobarbital, and caffeine in zolpidem-trained humans.**
  Author(s): Department of Psychiatry, University of Mississippi Medical Center, USA. crush2@pop.uky.edu
  Source: Rush, C R Baker, R W Rowlett, J K Exp-Clin-Psychopharmacol. 2000 February; 8(1): 22-36 1064-1297

- **Effect of the benzodiazepine receptor agonist, zolpidem, on palatable fluid consumption in the rat.**
  Author(s): Merck Sharp and Dohme Research Laboratories, Neuroscience Research Centre, Harlow, UK.
  Source: Stanhope, K J Roe, S Dawson, G Draper, F Jackson, A Psychopharmacology-(Berl). 1993; 111(2): 185-9 0033-3158

- **Effectiveness and tolerability of melatonin and zolpidem for the alleviation of jet lag.**
  Author(s): University of Zurich Travel Clinic, Switzerland.
  Source: Suhner, A Schlagenhauf, P Hofer, I Johnson, R Tschopp, A Steffen, R Aviat-Space-Environ-Med. 2001 July; 72(7): 638-46 0095-6562

- **Effects of alprazolam, caffeine, and zolpidem in humans trained to discriminate triazolam from placebo.**
  Author(s): Departments of Psychiatry and Psychology, University of Vermont, Burlington, VT 05401, USA. brandi@jhmi.edu
  Source: Smith, B J Bickel, W K Drug-Alcohol-Depend. 2001 February 1; 61(3): 249-60 0376-8716

- **GABA(A) receptor alpha-1 subunit deletion alters receptor subtype assembly, pharmacological and behavioral responses to benzodiazepines and zolpidem.**
  Author(s): Department of Pharmacology, University of North Carolina at Chapel Hill, 27599, USA.
  Source: Kralic, J E O'Buckley, T K Khisti, R T Hodge, C W Homanics, G E Morrow, A L Neuropharmacology. 2002 September; 43(4): 685-94 0028-3908

- **Hallucinations and Zolpidem.**
  Source: Anonymous Prescrire-Int. 2002 August; 11(60): 117 1167-7422

- **Prenatal exposure to diazepam and alprazolam, but not to zolpidem, affects behavioural stress reactivity in handling-naive and handling-habituated adult male rat progeny.**
  Author(s): Department of Pharmacological Sciences, Palermo University, V. Vespro 129, 90127 Palermo, Italy. psycho@unipa.it
  Source: Cannizzaro, C Martire, M Steardo, L Cannizzaro, E Gagliano, M Mineo, A Provenzano, G Brain-Res. 2002 October 25; 953(1-2): 170-80 0006-8993

- **The activity of zolpidem and other hypnotics within the gamma-aminobutyric acid (GABAA) receptor supramolecular complex, as determined by 35S-t-butylbicyclophosphorothionate (35S-TBPS) binding to rat cerebral cortex membranes.**
  Author(s): Synthelabo Recherche (L.E.R.S.), Bagneux, France.
  Source: Lloyd, G K Danielou, G Thuret, F J-Pharmacol-Exp-Ther. 1990 November; 255(2): 690-6 0022-3565

- **The effect of zolpidem on operant behavior and its relation to pharmacokinetics after intravenous and subcutaneous administration: concentration-effect relations.**
  Author(s): Rutgers, The State University of New Jersey, Piscataway, NJ, USA. celau@yahoo.com
  Source: Lau, C E Sun, L Wang, Q Falk, J L Behav-Pharmacol. 2002 March; 13(2): 93-103 0955-8810

- **The effects of diazepam and zolpidem on cocaine- and amphetamine-induced place preference.**
  Author(s): National Public Health Institute, Department of Mental Health and Alcohol Research, Helsinki, Finland.
  Source: Meririnne, E Kankaanpaa, A Lillsunde, P Seppala, T Pharmacol-Biochem-Behavolume 1999 January; 62(1): 159-64 0091-3057

- **Zinc and zolpidem modulate mIPSCs in rat neocortical pyramidal neurons.**
  Author(s): Department of Neurobiology, University of Alabama at Birmingham, Birmingham, Alabama 35294, USA.
  Source: Defazio, T Hablitz, J J J-Neurophysiol. 1998 October; 80(4): 1670-7 0022-3077

- **Zolpidem 10 mg given at daytime is not antagonized by 300 mg caffeine in man.**
  Author(s): Department of Pharmacology and Toxicology, Institute of Biomedicine, University of Helsinki, Finland.
  Source: Mattila, M J Nurminen, M L Vainio, P Vanakoski, J Eur-J-Clin-Pharmacol. 1998 July; 54(5): 421-5 0031-6970

- **Zolpidem and alpidem: two imidazopyridines with selectivity for omega 1- and omega 3-receptor subtypes.**
  Author(s): Department of Biology, Synthelabo Recherche (L.E.R.S.), Paris, France.
  Source: Langer, S Z Arbilla, S Benavides, J Scatton, B Adv-Biochem-Psychopharmacol. 1990; 4661-72 0065-2229

- **Zolpidem and driving impairment.**
  Author(s): State toxicologist, Bureau of Forensic Laboratory Services, Washington State Patrol, Seattle 89134, USA. blogan@wsp.wa.gov
  Source: Logan, B K Couper, F J J-Forensic-Sci. 2001 January; 46(1): 105-10 0022-1198

- **Zolpidem behavioral pharmacology in baboons: self-injection, discrimination, tolerance and withdrawal.**
  Author(s): Department of Psychiatry and Behavioral Sciences, Johns Hopkins University School of Medicine, Baltimore, Maryland.
  Source: Griffiths, R R Sannerud, C A Ator, N A Brady, J V J-Pharmacol-Exp-Ther. 1992 March; 260(3): 1199-208 0022-3565

- **Zolpidem in restless legs syndrome.**
  Author(s): Sleep Disorders Center, Department of Neurology, Universidade Estacio de Sa, Rio de Janeiro, Brazil.
  Source: Bezerra, M L Martinez, J V Eur-Neurol. 2002; 48(3): 180-1 0014-3022

Federal Resources on Nutrition

In addition to the IBIDS, the United States Department of Health and Human Services (HHS) and the United States Department of Agriculture (USDA) provide many sources of information on general nutrition and health. Recommended resources include:

- healthfinder®, HHS's gateway to health information, including diet and nutrition: **http://www.healthfinder.gov/scripts/SearchContext.asp?topic=238&page=0**

- The United States Department of Agriculture's Web site dedicated to nutrition information: **www.nutrition.gov**

- The Food and Drug Administration's Web site for federal food safety information: **www.foodsafety.gov**

- The National Action Plan on Overweight and Obesity sponsored by the United States Surgeon General: **http://www.surgeongeneral.gov/topics/obesity/**

- The Center for Food Safety and Applied Nutrition has an Internet site sponsored by the Food and Drug Administration and the Department of Health and Human Services: **http://vm.cfsan.fda.gov/**

- Center for Nutrition Policy and Promotion sponsored by the United States Department of Agriculture: **http://www.usda.gov/cnpp/**

- Food and Nutrition Information Center, National Agricultural Library sponsored by the United States Department of Agriculture: **http://www.nal.usda.gov/fnic/**

- Food and Nutrition Service sponsored by the United States Department of Agriculture: **http://www.fns.usda.gov/fns/**

Additional Web Resources

A number of additional Web sites offer encyclopedic information covering food and nutrition. The following is a representative sample:

- AOL: **http://search.aol.com/cat.adp?id=174&layer=&from=subcats**
- Family Village: **http://www.familyvillage.wisc.edu/med_nutrition.html**
- Google: **http://directory.google.com/Top/Health/Nutrition/**
- Healthnotes: **http://www.healthnotes.com/**
- Open Directory Project: **http://dmoz.org/Health/Nutrition/**
- Yahoo.com: **http://dir.yahoo.com/Health/Nutrition/**
- WebMD®Health: **http://my.webmd.com/nutrition**
- WholeHealthMD.com: **http://www.wholehealthmd.com/reflib/0,1529,00.html**

CHAPTER 3. ALTERNATIVE MEDICINE AND AMBIEN

Overview

In this chapter, we will begin by introducing you to official information sources on complementary and alternative medicine (CAM) relating to Ambien. At the conclusion of this chapter, we will provide additional sources.

National Center for Complementary and Alternative Medicine

The National Center for Complementary and Alternative Medicine (NCCAM) of the National Institutes of Health (http://nccam.nih.gov/) has created a link to the National Library of Medicine's databases to facilitate research for articles that specifically relate to Ambien and complementary medicine. To search the database, go to the following Web site: **http://www.nlm.nih.gov/nccam/camonpubmed.html**. Select "CAM on PubMed." Enter "Ambien" (or synonyms) into the search box. Click "Go." The following references provide information on particular aspects of complementary and alternative medicine that are related to Ambien:

- **Assessment of a new hypnotic imidazo-pyridine (zolpidem) as oral premedication.**
  Author(s): Cashman JN, Power SJ, Jones RM.
  Source: British Journal of Clinical Pharmacology. 1987 July; 24(1): 85-92.
  http://www.ncbi.nlm.nih.gov:80/entrez/query.fcgi?cmd=Retrieve&db=PubMed&list_uids=2887188&dopt=Abstract

- **Beyond benzodiazepines: alternative pharmacologic agents for the treatment of insomnia.**
  Author(s): Wagner J, Wagner ML, Hening WA.
  Source: The Annals of Pharmacotherapy. 1998 June; 32(6): 680-91. Review.
  http://www.ncbi.nlm.nih.gov:80/entrez/query.fcgi?cmd=Retrieve&db=PubMed&list_uids=9640488&dopt=Abstract

- **Extraordinary arousal from semi-comatose state on zolpidem. A case report.**
  Author(s): Clauss RP, Guldenpfennig WM, Nel HW, Sathekge MM, Venkannagari RR.

Source: South African Medical Journal. Suid-Afrikaanse Tydskrif Vir Geneeskunde. 2000 January; 90(1): 68-72.
http://www.ncbi.nlm.nih.gov:80/entrez/query.fcgi?cmd=Retrieve&db=PubMed&list_uids=10721397&dopt=Abstract

- **Functional neuroanatomy of human sleep states after zolpidem and placebo: a H215O-PET study.**
  Author(s): Finelli LA, Landolt HP, Buck A, Roth C, Berthold T, Borbely AA, Achermann P.
  Source: Journal of Sleep Research. 2000 June; 9(2): 161-73.
  http://www.ncbi.nlm.nih.gov:80/entrez/query.fcgi?cmd=Retrieve&db=PubMed&list_uids=10849243&dopt=Abstract

- **Pathophysiology and management of insomnia during depression.**
  Author(s): Kupfer DJ.
  Source: Annals of Clinical Psychiatry : Official Journal of the American Academy of Clinical Psychiatrists. 1999 December; 11(4): 267-76. Review.
  http://www.ncbi.nlm.nih.gov:80/entrez/query.fcgi?cmd=Retrieve&db=PubMed&list_uids=10596741&dopt=Abstract

- **Zolpidem and sleep deprivation: different effect on EEG power spectra.**
  Author(s): Landolt HP, Finelli LA, Roth C, Buck A, Achermann P, Borbely AA.
  Source: Journal of Sleep Research. 2000 June; 9(2): 175-83.
  http://www.ncbi.nlm.nih.gov:80/entrez/query.fcgi?cmd=Retrieve&db=PubMed&list_uids=10849244&dopt=Abstract

Additional Web Resources

A number of additional Web sites offer encyclopedic information covering CAM and related topics. The following is a representative sample:

- Alternative Medicine Foundation, Inc.: **http://www.herbmed.org/**
- AOL: **http://search.aol.com/cat.adp?id=169&layer=&from=subcats**
- Chinese Medicine: **http://www.newcenturynutrition.com/**
- drkoop.com®: **http://www.drkoop.com/InteractiveMedicine/IndexC.html**
- Family Village: **http://www.familyvillage.wisc.edu/med_altn.htm**
- Google: **http://directory.google.com/Top/Health/Alternative/**
- Healthnotes: **http://www.healthnotes.com/**
- MedWebPlus: **http://medwebplus.com/subject/Alternative_and_Complementary_Medicine**
- Open Directory Project: **http://dmoz.org/Health/Alternative/**
- HealthGate: **http://www.tnp.com/**
- WebMD®Health: **http://my.webmd.com/drugs_and_herbs**
- WholeHealthMD.com: **http://www.wholehealthmd.com/reflib/0,1529,00.html**

- Yahoo.com: **http://dir.yahoo.com/Health/Alternative_Medicine/**

The following is a specific Web list relating to Ambien; please note that any particular subject below may indicate either a therapeutic use, or a contraindication (potential danger), and does not reflect an official recommendation:

- **General Overview**

    Insomnia
    Source: Healthnotes, Inc.; www.healthnotes.com

    Insomnia
    Source: Prima Communications, Inc.www.personalhealthzone.com

- **Herbs and Supplements**

    5-htp
    Alternative names: 5-Hydroxytryptophan (5-HTP)
    Source: Integrative Medicine Communications; www.drkoop.com

    5-hydroxytryptophan
    Source: Healthnotes, Inc.; www.healthnotes.com

    5-hydroxytryptophan (5-htp)
    Alternative names: 5-HTP
    Source: Integrative Medicine Communications; www.drkoop.com

    English Lavendar
    Source: Integrative Medicine Communications; www.drkoop.com

    French Lavendar
    Source: Integrative Medicine Communications; www.drkoop.com

    Lavandula Angustifolia
    Source: Integrative Medicine Communications; www.drkoop.com

    Lavender
    Alternative names: Lavandula officinalis
    Source: Healthnotes, Inc.; www.healthnotes.com

    Lavender
    Alternative names: Lavandula angustifolia, English Lavendar, French Lavendar
    Source: Integrative Medicine Communications; www.drkoop.com

    Valerian
    Source: Prima Communications, Inc.www.personalhealthzone.com

    Zolpidem
    Source: Healthnotes, Inc.; www.healthnotes.com

General References

A good place to find general background information on CAM is the National Library of Medicine. It has prepared within the MEDLINEplus system an information topic page dedicated to complementary and alternative medicine. To access this page, go to the MEDLINEplus site at **http://www.nlm.nih.gov/medlineplus/alternativemedicine.html** This Web site provides a general overview of various topics and can lead to a number of general sources.

CHAPTER 4. PATENTS ON AMBIEN

Overview

Patents can be physical innovations (e.g. chemicals, pharmaceuticals, medical equipment) or processes (e.g. treatments or diagnostic procedures). The United States Patent and Trademark Office defines a patent as a grant of a property right to the inventor, issued by the Patent and Trademark Office.[8] Patents, therefore, are intellectual property. For the United States, the term of a new patent is 20 years from the date when the patent application was filed. If the inventor wishes to receive economic benefits, it is likely that the invention will become commercially available within 20 years of the initial filing. It is important to understand, therefore, that an inventor's patent does not indicate that a product or service is or will be commercially available. The patent implies only that the inventor has "the right to exclude others from making, using, offering for sale, or selling" the invention in the United States. While this relates to U.S. patents, similar rules govern foreign patents.

In this chapter, we show you how to locate information on patents and their inventors. If you find a patent that is particularly interesting to you, contact the inventor or the assignee for further information. **IMPORTANT NOTE:** When following the search strategy described below, you may discover non-medical patents that use the generic term "Ambien" (or a synonym) in their titles. To accurately reflect the results that you might find while conducting research on Ambien, we have not necessarily excluded non-medical patents in this bibliography.

Patents on Ambien

By performing a patent search focusing on Ambien, you can obtain information such as the title of the invention, the names of the inventor(s), the assignee(s) or the company that owns or controls the patent, a short abstract that summarizes the patent, and a few excerpts from the description of the patent. The abstract of a patent tends to be more technical in nature, while the description is often written for the public. Full patent descriptions contain much more information than is presented here (e.g. claims, references, figures, diagrams, etc.). We

---

[8] Adapted from the United States Patent and Trademark Office: http://www.uspto.gov/web/offices/pac/doc/general/whatis.htm.

will tell you how to obtain this information later in the chapter. The following is an example of the type of information that you can expect to obtain from a patent search on Ambien:

- **Controlled-release dosage forms comprising zolpidem or a salt thereof**

    Inventor(s): Alaux; Gerard (Beynes, FR), Andre; Frederic (Antony, FR), Lewis; Gareth (Dourdan, FR)

    Assignee(s): Sanofi-Synthelabo (Paris, FR)

    Patent Number: 6,514,531

    Date filed: July 16, 2001

    Abstract: The present invention relates to controlled-release dosage forms of zolpidem or salts thereof adapted to release zolpidem over a predetermined time period, according to a biphasic profile of dissolution, where the first phase is an immediate release phase and the second phase is a prolonged release phase and particular embodiments thereof intended to avoid abuse.

    Excerpt(s): The present invention relates to controlled-release dosage forms comprising zolpidem or salts thereof. Zolpidem is a suitable short acting hypnotic for the controlled-release dosage form according to the present invention. Zolpidem is a hypnotic from the therapeutical class of imidazopyridines. It is administrated orally by means of a tablet or other solid dosage form. Zolpidem acts rapidly. Indeed pharmacokinetic and pharmacodynamic data show that zolpidem has both a rapid absorption and onset of hypnotic action. Its bioavailability is 70% following oral administration and demonstrates linear kinetics in the therapeutic dose range, which lies between 5 and 10 mg in conventional forms, peak plasma concentration is reached at between 0.5 and 3 hours, the elimination half-life is short, with a mean of 2.4 hours and a duration of action of up to 6 hours. For reasons of simplicity, in the absence of contrary indication, within the whole description "zolpidem" or the "drug" means zolpidem per se as well as its salts. The preferred salt of zolpidem is zolpidem hemitartrate.

    Web site: http://www.delphion.com/details?pn=US06514531__

- **Zolpidem salt forms**

    Inventor(s): Lemmens; Jacobus Maria (Mook, NL), Peters; Theodorus Hendricus Antonius (Arnhem, NL), Picha; Frantisek (Brno, CZ), Ettema; Gerrit Jan Bouke (Denekamp, NL)

    Assignee(s): Synthon BV (NL)

    Patent Number: 6,242,460

    Date filed: November 26, 1999

    Abstract: Zolpidem salts having improved physical stability do not exhibit a melting endotherm corresponding to zolpidem free base when heated at 5.degree. C./minute from about 25.degree. C. to 250.degree. C. The salts are generally easy to reproduce, even on an industrial scale and are easier to handle due to the increased stability than the known zolpidem tartrate. The zolpidem salts are typically pharmaceutically acceptable salts and can be used in formulating pharmaceutical compositions and in pharmaceutical uses; e.g. as a hypnotic.

Excerpt(s): The present invention relates to novel salt forms of zolpidem and to pharmaceutical compositions and methods of treatment containing the same. It has been marketed in solid dosage forms for peroral application (tablets) under the trade marks AMBIEN.RTM. and STILNOX.RTM. As the active substance in these pharmaceutical dosage forms, zolpidem is present in the form of a salt with natural L(+)tartaric acid ((2R,3R)-2,3-dihydroxybutanedicarboxylic acid) wherein the molar ratio of zolpidem and tartaric acid in the salt is 2:1. This salt is conventionally called zolpidem hemitartrate but more a correct denomination thereof, which will be used hereinafter, is zolpidem tartrate. The zolpidem free base was disclosed generically in EP 50563 of Synthelabo. The zolpidem tartrate used in the commercial products, along with an improved synthesis scheme, was subsequently disclosed in EP 251859 (U.S. Pat. No. 4,794,185). It is believed that the process set forth in this patent corresponds to the commercial process presently used for the production of zolpidem. An example therein shows the production of zolpidem and the formation of the tartrate salt. Specifically, 25 g of zolpidem free base is dissolved in 180 ml of methanol and combined with 60 ml of a methanol solution containing 6.1 g of tartaric acid (a 1:2 molar ratio) and then allowing the mixed solution to crystallize. The crystalline product is reported to have a melting point of 197.degree. C. The specific details of how the crystallization is performed are not disclosed.

Web site: http://www.delphion.com/details?pn=US06242460__

Patent Applications on Ambien

As of December 2000, U.S. patent applications are open to public viewing.[9] Applications are patent requests which have yet to be granted. (The process to achieve a patent can take several years.) The following patent applications have been filed since December 2000 relating to Ambien:

- **Zolpidem hemitartrate**

    Inventor(s): Aronhime, Judith; (Rechovot, IL), Leonov, David; (Rechovot, IL), Meszaros-Sos, Erzebet; (Debrecen, HU), Salyi, Szaboles; (Debrecen, HU), Szabo, Csaba; (Debrecen, HU), Zavurov, Shlomo; (Lod, IL)

    Correspondence: KENYON & KENYON; ONE BROADWAY; NEW YORK; NY; 10004; US

    Patent Application Number: 20020077332

    Date filed: April 24, 2001

    Abstract: The present invention provides for novel polymorphs of zolpidem hemitartrate and the preparation of the polymorphs.

    Excerpt(s): This invention claims the benefit under 35 U.S.C. 1.119(e) of provisional applications Serial No. 60/199,298, filed Apr. 24, 2000; No. 60/206,025, filed May 2, 2000 and No. 60/225,364, filed Aug. 14, 2000. The present invention relates to novel hydrate, anhydrous and solvate crystal forms of zolpidem hemitartrate and the preparation thereof. Zolpidem, as a hemitartrate salt, is currently approved for the short-term treatment of insomnia in the United States under the trademark of AMBIEN. Zolpidem hemitartrate is classified as a non-benzodiazepine hypnotic of the imidazopyridine

---

[9] This has been a common practice outside the United States prior to December 2000.

class. It has little effect on the stages of sleep in normal human subjects and is as effective as benzodiazepines in shortening sleep latency and prolonging total sleep time in patients with insomnia. The development of tolerance and physical dependence for patients using AMBIEN has been seen only very rarely and under unusual circumstances. (Goodman and Gilman's, The Pharmacological Basis of Therapeutics 371 (Joel G. Hardman et al., eds. 9th ed. 1996)).

Web site: http://appft1.uspto.gov/netahtml/PTO/search-bool.html

Keeping Current

In order to stay informed about patents and patent applications dealing with Ambien, you can access the U.S. Patent Office archive via the Internet at the following Web address: **http://www.uspto.gov/patft/index.html**. You will see two broad options: (1) Issued Patent, and (2) Published Applications. To see a list of issued patents, perform the following steps: Under "Issued Patents," click "Quick Search." Then, type "Ambien" (or synonyms) into the "Term 1" box. After clicking on the search button, scroll down to see the various patents which have been granted to date on Ambien.

You can also use this procedure to view pending patent applications concerning Ambien. Simply go back to **http://www.uspto.gov/patft/index.html**. Select "Quick Search" under "Published Applications." Then proceed with the steps listed above.

CHAPTER 5. PERIODICALS AND NEWS ON AMBIEN

Overview

In this chapter, we suggest a number of news sources and present various periodicals that cover Ambien.

News Services and Press Releases

One of the simplest ways of tracking press releases on Ambien is to search the news wires. In the following sample of sources, we will briefly describe how to access each service. These services only post recent news intended for public viewing.

PR Newswire

To access the PR Newswire archive, simply go to **http://www.prnewswire.com/**. Select your country. Type "Ambien" (or synonyms) into the search box. You will automatically receive information on relevant news releases posted within the last 30 days. The search results are shown by order of relevance.

Reuters Health

The Reuters' Medical News and Health eLine databases can be very useful in exploring news archives relating to Ambien. While some of the listed articles are free to view, others are available for purchase for a nominal fee. To access this archive, go to **http://www.reutershealth.com/en/index.html** and search by "Ambien" (or synonyms). The following was recently listed in this archive for Ambien:

- **FDA tentatively approves Biovail's rapid-dissolving zolpidem**
  Source: Reuters Industry Breifing
  Date: November 01, 2002

- **Biovail files NDA for orally-dissolving version of Ambien**
  Source: Reuters Industry Breifing
  Date: January 10, 2002

- **Zolpidem Effective In Short-Term Treatment Of Chronic Insomnia**
  Source: Reuters Medical News
  Date: April 04, 1997

The NIH

Within MEDLINEplus, the NIH has made an agreement with the New York Times Syndicate, the AP News Service, and Reuters to deliver news that can be browsed by the public. Search news releases at **http://www.nlm.nih.gov/medlineplus/alphanews_a.html**. MEDLINEplus allows you to browse across an alphabetical index. Or you can search by date at the following Web page: **http://www.nlm.nih.gov/medlineplus/newsbydate.html**. Often, news items are indexed by MEDLINEplus within its search engine.

Business Wire

Business Wire is similar to PR Newswire. To access this archive, simply go to **http://www.businesswire.com/**. You can scan the news by industry category or company name.

Market Wire

Market Wire is more focused on technology than the other wires. To browse the latest press releases by topic, such as alternative medicine, biotechnology, fitness, healthcare, legal, nutrition, and pharmaceuticals, access Market Wire's Medical/Health channel at **http://www.marketwire.com/mw/release_index?channel=MedicalHealth**. Or simply go to Market Wire's home page at **http://www.marketwire.com/mw/home**, type "Ambien" (or synonyms) into the search box, and click on "Search News." As this service is technology oriented, you may wish to use it when searching for press releases covering diagnostic procedures or tests.

Search Engines

Medical news is also available in the news sections of commercial Internet search engines. See the health news page at Yahoo (**http://dir.yahoo.com/Health/News_and_Media/**), or you can use this Web site's general news search page at **http://news.yahoo.com/**. Type in "Ambien" (or synonyms). If you know the name of a company that is relevant to Ambien, you can go to any stock trading Web site (such as **http://www.etrade.com/**) and search for the company name there. News items across various news sources are reported on indicated hyperlinks. Google offers a similar service at **http://news.google.com/**.

BBC

Covering news from a more European perspective, the British Broadcasting Corporation (BBC) allows the public free access to their news archive located at **http://www.bbc.co.uk/**. Search by "Ambien" (or synonyms).

Academic Periodicals covering Ambien

Numerous periodicals are currently indexed within the National Library of Medicine's PubMed database that are known to publish articles relating to Ambien. In addition to these sources, you can search for articles covering Ambien that have been published by any of the periodicals listed in previous chapters. To find the latest studies published, go to **http://www.ncbi.nlm.nih.gov/pubmed**, type the name of the periodical into the search box, and click "Go."

If you want complete details about the historical contents of a journal, you can also visit the following Web site: **http://www.ncbi.nlm.nih.gov/entrez/jrbrowser.cgi**. Here, type in the name of the journal or its abbreviation, and you will receive an index of published articles. At **http://locatorplus.gov/**, you can retrieve more indexing information on medical periodicals (e.g. the name of the publisher). Select the button "Search LOCATORplus." Then type in the name of the journal and select the advanced search option "Journal Title Search."

CHAPTER 6. RESEARCHING MEDICATIONS

Overview

While a number of hard copy or CD-ROM resources are available for researching medications, a more flexible method is to use Internet-based databases. Broadly speaking, there are two sources of information on approved medications: public sources and private sources. We will emphasize free-to-use public sources.

U.S. Pharmacopeia

Because of historical investments by various organizations and the emergence of the Internet, it has become rather simple to learn about the medications recommended for Ambien. One such source is the United States Pharmacopeia. In 1820, eleven physicians met in Washington, D.C. to establish the first compendium of standard drugs for the United States. They called this compendium the U.S. Pharmacopeia (USP). Today, the USP is a non-profit organization consisting of 800 volunteer scientists, eleven elected officials, and 400 representatives of state associations and colleges of medicine and pharmacy. The USP is located in Rockville, Maryland, and its home page is located at **http://www.usp.org/**. The USP currently provides standards for over 3,700 medications. The resulting USP DI® Advice for the Patient® can be accessed through the National Library of Medicine of the National Institutes of Health. The database is partially derived from lists of federally approved medications in the Food and Drug Administration's (FDA) Drug Approvals database, located at **http://www.fda.gov/cder/da/da.htm**.

While the FDA database is rather large and difficult to navigate, the Phamacopeia is both user-friendly and free to use. It covers more than 9,000 prescription and over-the-counter medications. To access this database, simply type the following hyperlink into your Web browser: **http://www.nlm.nih.gov/medlineplus/druginformation.html**. To view examples of a given medication (brand names, category, description, preparation, proper use, precautions, side effects, etc.), simply follow the hyperlinks indicated within the United States Pharmacopeia (USP).

Below, we have compiled a list of medications associated with Ambien. If you would like more information on a particular medication, the provided hyperlinks will direct you to ample documentation (e.g. typical dosage, side effects, drug-interaction risks, etc.). The following drugs have been mentioned in the Pharmacopeia and other sources as being potentially applicable to Ambien:

Zolpidem
- **Systemic - U.S. Brands:** Ambien
  http://www.nlm.nih.gov/medlineplus/druginfo/uspdi/202707.html

Commercial Databases

In addition to the medications listed in the USP above, a number of commercial sites are available by subscription to physicians and their institutions. Or, you may be able to access these sources from your local medical library.

Mosby's Drug Consult™

Mosby's Drug Consult™ database (also available on CD-ROM and book format) covers 45,000 drug products including generics and international brands. It provides prescribing information, drug interactions, and patient information. Subscription information is available at the following hyperlink: **http://www.mosbysdrugconsult.com/**.

PDR*health*

The PDR*health* database is a free-to-use, drug information search engine that has been written for the public in layman's terms. It contains FDA-approved drug information adapted from the Physicians' Desk Reference (PDR) database. PDR*health* can be searched by brand name, generic name, or indication. It features multiple drug interactions reports. Search PDR*health* at **http://www.pdrhealth.com/drug_info/index.html**.

Other Web Sites

Drugs.com (**www.drugs.com**) reproduces the information in the Pharmacopeia as well as commercial information. You may also want to consider the Web site of the Medical Letter, Inc. (**http://www.medletter.com/**) which allows users to download articles on various drugs and therapeutics for a nominal fee.

Researching Orphan Drugs

Although the list of orphan drugs is revised on a daily basis, you can quickly research orphan drugs that might be applicable to Ambien by using the database managed by the National Organization for Rare Disorders, Inc. (NORD), at **http://www.rarediseases.org/**. Scroll down the page, and on the left toolbar, click on "Orphan Drug Designation Database." On this page (**http://www.rarediseases.org/search/noddsearch.html**), type "Ambien" (or synonyms) into the search box, and click "Submit Query." When you receive your results, note that not all of the drugs may be relevant, as some may have been withdrawn from orphan status. Write down or print out the name of each drug and the relevant contact information. From there, visit the Pharmacopeia Web site and type the name of each orphan drug into the search box at **http://www.nlm.nih.gov/medlineplus/druginformation.html** You may need to contact the sponsor or NORD for further information.

NORD conducts "early access programs for investigational new drugs (IND) under the Food and Drug Administration's (FDA's) approval 'Treatment INDs' programs which allow for a limited number of individuals to receive investigational drugs before FDA marketing approval." If the orphan product about which you are seeking information is approved for marketing, information on side effects can be found on the product's label. If the product is not approved, you may need to contact the sponsor.

The following is a list of orphan drugs currently listed in the NORD Orphan Drug Designation Database for Ambien:

- **Eflornithine HCI (trade name: Ornidyl)**

    http://www.rarediseases.org/nord/search/nodd_full?code=313

If you have any questions about a medical treatment, the FDA may have an office near you. Look for their number in the blue pages of the phone book. You can also contact the FDA through its toll-free number, 1-888-INFO-FDA (1-888-463-6332), or on the World Wide Web at **www.fda.gov**.

APPENDICES

APPENDIX A. PHYSICIAN RESOURCES

Overview

In this chapter, we focus on databases and Internet-based guidelines and information resources created or written for a professional audience.

NIH Guidelines

Commonly referred to as "clinical" or "professional" guidelines, the National Institutes of Health publish physician guidelines for the most common diseases. Publications are available at the following by relevant Institute[10]:

- Office of the Director (OD); guidelines consolidated across agencies available at
  http://www.nih.gov/health/consumer/conkey.htm

- National Institute of General Medical Sciences (NIGMS); fact sheets available at
  http://www.nigms.nih.gov/news/facts/

- National Library of Medicine (NLM); extensive encyclopedia (A.D.A.M., Inc.) with guidelines: http://www.nlm.nih.gov/medlineplus/healthtopics.html

- National Cancer Institute (NCI); guidelines available at
  http://www.cancer.gov/cancerinfo/list.aspx?viewid=5f35036e-5497-4d86-8c2c-714a9f7c8d25

- National Eye Institute (NEI); guidelines available at
  http://www.nei.nih.gov/order/index.htm

- National Heart, Lung, and Blood Institute (NHLBI); guidelines available at
  http://www.nhlbi.nih.gov/guidelines/index.htm

- National Human Genome Research Institute (NHGRI); research available at
  http://www.genome.gov/page.cfm?pageID=10000375

- National Institute on Aging (NIA); guidelines available at
  http://www.nia.nih.gov/health/

---

[10] These publications are typically written by one or more of the various NIH Institutes.

- National Institute on Alcohol Abuse and Alcoholism (NIAAA); guidelines available at **http://www.niaaa.nih.gov/publications/publications.htm**

- National Institute of Allergy and Infectious Diseases (NIAID); guidelines available at **http://www.niaid.nih.gov/publications/**

- National Institute of Arthritis and Musculoskeletal and Skin Diseases (NIAMS); fact sheets and guidelines available at **http://www.niams.nih.gov/hi/index.htm**

- National Institute of Child Health and Human Development (NICHD); guidelines available at **http://www.nichd.nih.gov/publications/pubskey.cfm**

- National Institute on Deafness and Other Communication Disorders (NIDCD); fact sheets and guidelines at **http://www.nidcd.nih.gov/health/**

- National Institute of Dental and Craniofacial Research (NIDCR); guidelines available at **http://www.nidr.nih.gov/health/**

- National Institute of Diabetes and Digestive and Kidney Diseases (NIDDK); guidelines available at **http://www.niddk.nih.gov/health/health.htm**

- National Institute on Drug Abuse (NIDA); guidelines available at **http://www.nida.nih.gov/DrugAbuse.html**

- National Institute of Environmental Health Sciences (NIEHS); environmental health information available at **http://www.niehs.nih.gov/external/facts.htm**

- National Institute of Mental Health (NIMH); guidelines available at **http://www.nimh.nih.gov/practitioners/index.cfm**

- National Institute of Neurological Disorders and Stroke (NINDS); neurological disorder information pages available at **http://www.ninds.nih.gov/health_and_medical/disorder_index.htm**

- National Institute of Nursing Research (NINR); publications on selected illnesses at **http://www.nih.gov/ninr/news-info/publications.html**

- National Institute of Biomedical Imaging and Bioengineering; general information at **http://grants.nih.gov/grants/becon/becon_info.htm**

- Center for Information Technology (CIT); referrals to other agencies based on keyword searches available at **http://kb.nih.gov/www_query_main.asp**

- National Center for Complementary and Alternative Medicine (NCCAM); health information available at **http://nccam.nih.gov/health/**

- National Center for Research Resources (NCRR); various information directories available at **http://www.ncrr.nih.gov/publications.asp**

- Office of Rare Diseases; various fact sheets available at **http://rarediseases.info.nih.gov/html/resources/rep_pubs.html**

- Centers for Disease Control and Prevention; various fact sheets on infectious diseases available at **http://www.cdc.gov/publications.htm**

NIH Databases

In addition to the various Institutes of Health that publish professional guidelines, the NIH has designed a number of databases for professionals.[11] Physician-oriented resources provide a wide variety of information related to the biomedical and health sciences, both past and present. The format of these resources varies. Searchable databases, bibliographic citations, full-text articles (when available), archival collections, and images are all available. The following are referenced by the National Library of Medicine:[12]

- **Bioethics:** Access to published literature on the ethical, legal, and public policy issues surrounding healthcare and biomedical research. This information is provided in conjunction with the Kennedy Institute of Ethics located at Georgetown University, Washington, D.C.: http://www.nlm.nih.gov/databases/databases_bioethics.html

- **HIV/AIDS Resources:** Describes various links and databases dedicated to HIV/AIDS research: http://www.nlm.nih.gov/pubs/factsheets/aidsinfs.html

- **NLM Online Exhibitions:** Describes "Exhibitions in the History of Medicine": http://www.nlm.nih.gov/exhibition/exhibition.html. Additional resources for historical scholarship in medicine: http://www.nlm.nih.gov/hmd/hmd.html

- **Biotechnology Information:** Access to public databases. The National Center for Biotechnology Information conducts research in computational biology, develops software tools for analyzing genome data, and disseminates biomedical information for the better understanding of molecular processes affecting human health and disease: http://www.ncbi.nlm.nih.gov/

- **Population Information:** The National Library of Medicine provides access to worldwide coverage of population, family planning, and related health issues, including family planning technology and programs, fertility, and population law and policy: http://www.nlm.nih.gov/databases/databases_population.html

- **Cancer Information:** Access to cancer-oriented databases: http://www.nlm.nih.gov/databases/databases_cancer.html

- **Profiles in Science:** Offering the archival collections of prominent twentieth-century biomedical scientists to the public through modern digital technology: http://www.profiles.nlm.nih.gov/

- **Chemical Information:** Provides links to various chemical databases and references: http://sis.nlm.nih.gov/Chem/ChemMain.html

- **Clinical Alerts:** Reports the release of findings from the NIH-funded clinical trials where such release could significantly affect morbidity and mortality: http://www.nlm.nih.gov/databases/alerts/clinical_alerts.html

- **Space Life Sciences:** Provides links and information to space-based research (including NASA): http://www.nlm.nih.gov/databases/databases_space.html

- **MEDLINE:** Bibliographic database covering the fields of medicine, nursing, dentistry, veterinary medicine, the healthcare system, and the pre-clinical sciences: http://www.nlm.nih.gov/databases/databases_medline.html

---

[11] Remember, for the general public, the National Library of Medicine recommends the databases referenced in MEDLINE*plus* (http://medlineplus.gov/ or http://www.nlm.nih.gov/medlineplus/databases.html).

[12] See http://www.nlm.nih.gov/databases/databases.html.

- **Toxicology and Environmental Health Information (TOXNET):** Databases covering toxicology and environmental health: **http://sis.nlm.nih.gov/Tox/ToxMain.html**
- **Visible Human Interface:** Anatomically detailed, three-dimensional representations of normal male and female human bodies: **http://www.nlm.nih.gov/research/visible/visible_human.html**

The NLM Gateway[13]

The NLM (National Library of Medicine) Gateway is a Web-based system that lets users search simultaneously in multiple retrieval systems at the U.S. National Library of Medicine (NLM). It allows users of NLM services to initiate searches from one Web interface, providing one-stop searching for many of NLM's information resources or databases.[14] To use the NLM Gateway, simply go to the search site at **http://gateway.nlm.nih.gov/gw/Cmd**. Type "Ambien" (or synonyms) into the search box and click "Search." The results will be presented in a tabular form, indicating the number of references in each database category.

Results Summary

Category	Items Found
Journal Articles	556
Books / Periodicals / Audio Visual	0
Consumer Health	286
Meeting Abstracts	0
Other Collections	0
Total	842

HSTAT[15]

HSTAT is a free, Web-based resource that provides access to full-text documents used in healthcare decision-making.[16] These documents include clinical practice guidelines, quick-reference guides for clinicians, consumer health brochures, evidence reports and technology assessments from the Agency for Healthcare Research and Quality (AHRQ), as well as AHRQ's Put Prevention Into Practice.[17] Simply search by "Ambien" (or synonyms) at the following Web site: **http://text.nlm.nih.gov**.

---

[13] Adapted from NLM: **http://gateway.nlm.nih.gov/gw/Cmd?Overview.x**.

[14] The NLM Gateway is currently being developed by the Lister Hill National Center for Biomedical Communications (LHNCBC) at the National Library of Medicine (NLM) of the National Institutes of Health (NIH).

[15] Adapted from HSTAT: **http://www.nlm.nih.gov/pubs/factsheets/hstat.html**.

[16] The HSTAT URL is **http://hstat.nlm.nih.gov/**.

[17] Other important documents in HSTAT include: the National Institutes of Health (NIH) Consensus Conference Reports and Technology Assessment Reports; the HIV/AIDS Treatment Information Service (ATIS) resource documents; the Substance Abuse and Mental Health Services Administration's Center for Substance Abuse Treatment (SAMHSA/CSAT) Treatment Improvement Protocols (TIP) and Center for Substance Abuse Prevention (SAMHSA/CSAP) Prevention Enhancement Protocols System (PEPS); the Public Health Service (PHS) Preventive Services Task Force's *Guide to Clinical Preventive Services*; the independent, nonfederal Task Force on Community Services' *Guide to Community Preventive Services*; and the Health Technology Advisory Committee (HTAC) of the Minnesota Health Care Commission (MHCC) health technology evaluations.

Coffee Break: Tutorials for Biologists [18]

Coffee Break is a general healthcare site that takes a scientific view of the news and covers recent breakthroughs in biology that may one day assist physicians in developing treatments. Here you will find a collection of short reports on recent biological discoveries. Each report incorporates interactive tutorials that demonstrate how bioinformatics tools are used as a part of the research process. Currently, all Coffee Breaks are written by NCBI staff.[19] Each report is about 400 words and is usually based on a discovery reported in one or more articles from recently published, peer-reviewed literature.[20] This site has new articles every few weeks, so it can be considered an online magazine of sorts. It is intended for general background information. You can access the Coffee Break Web site at the following hyperlink: **http://www.ncbi.nlm.nih.gov/Coffeebreak/**.

Other Commercial Databases

In addition to resources maintained by official agencies, other databases exist that are commercial ventures addressing medical professionals. Here are some examples that may interest you:

- **CliniWeb International:** Index and table of contents to selected clinical information on the Internet; see **http://www.ohsu.edu/cliniweb/**.

- **Medical World Search:** Searches full text from thousands of selected medical sites on the Internet; see **http://www.mwsearch.com/**.

---

[18] Adapted from **http://www.ncbi.nlm.nih.gov/Coffeebreak/Archive/FAQ.html**.

[19] The figure that accompanies each article is frequently supplied by an expert external to NCBI, in which case the source of the figure is cited. The result is an interactive tutorial that tells a biological story.

[20] After a brief introduction that sets the work described into a broader context, the report focuses on how a molecular understanding can provide explanations of observed biology and lead to therapies for diseases. Each vignette is accompanied by a figure and hypertext links that lead to a series of pages that interactively show how NCBI tools and resources are used in the research process.

APPENDIX B. PATIENT RESOURCES

Overview

Official agencies, as well as federally funded institutions supported by national grants, frequently publish a variety of guidelines written with the patient in mind. These are typically called "Fact Sheets" or "Guidelines." They can take the form of a brochure, information kit, pamphlet, or flyer. Often they are only a few pages in length. Since new guidelines on Ambien can appear at any moment and be published by a number of sources, the best approach to finding guidelines is to systematically scan the Internet-based services that post them.

Patient Guideline Sources

The remainder of this chapter directs you to sources which either publish or can help you find additional guidelines on topics related to Ambien. Due to space limitations, these sources are listed in a concise manner. Do not hesitate to consult the following sources by either using the Internet hyperlink provided, or, in cases where the contact information is provided, contacting the publisher or author directly.

The National Institutes of Health

The NIH gateway to patients is located at **http://health.nih.gov/**. From this site, you can search across various sources and institutes, a number of which are summarized below.

Topic Pages: MEDLINEplus

The National Library of Medicine has created a vast and patient-oriented healthcare information portal called MEDLINEplus. Within this Internet-based system are "health topic pages" which list links to available materials relevant to Ambien. To access this system, log on to **http://www.nlm.nih.gov/medlineplus/healthtopics.html**. From there you can either search using the alphabetical index or browse by broad topic areas. Recently, MEDLINEplus listed the following when searched for "Ambien":

- Other guides

    Alzheimer's Disease
    http://www.nlm.nih.gov/medlineplus/alzheimersdisease.html

    Bipolar Disorder
    http://www.nlm.nih.gov/medlineplus/bipolardisorder.html

    Club Drugs
    http://www.nlm.nih.gov/medlineplus/clubdrugs.html

    Interstitial Cystitis
    http://www.nlm.nih.gov/medlineplus/interstitialcystitis.html

    Prescription Drug Abuse
    http://www.nlm.nih.gov/medlineplus/prescriptiondrugabuse.html

    Sleep Disorders
    http://www.nlm.nih.gov/medlineplus/sleepdisorders.html

You may also choose to use the search utility provided by MEDLINEplus at the following Web address: **http://www.nlm.nih.gov/medlineplus/**. Simply type a keyword into the search box and click "Search." This utility is similar to the NIH search utility, with the exception that it only includes materials that are linked within the MEDLINEplus system (mostly patient-oriented information). It also has the disadvantage of generating unstructured results. We recommend, therefore, that you use this method only if you have a very targeted search.

The NIH Search Utility

The NIH search utility allows you to search for documents on over 100 selected Web sites that comprise the NIH-WEB-SPACE. Each of these servers is "crawled" and indexed on an ongoing basis. Your search will produce a list of various documents, all of which will relate in some way to Ambien. The drawbacks of this approach are that the information is not organized by theme and that the references are often a mix of information for professionals and patients. Nevertheless, a large number of the listed Web sites provide useful background information. We can only recommend this route, therefore, for relatively rare or specific disorders, or when using highly targeted searches. To use the NIH search utility, visit the following Web page: **http://search.nih.gov/index.html**.

Additional Web Sources

A number of Web sites are available to the public that often link to government sites. These can also point you in the direction of essential information. The following is a representative sample:

- AOL: **http://search.aol.com/cat.adp?id=168&layer=&from=subcats**

- Family Village: **http://www.familyvillage.wisc.edu/specific.htm**

- Google: **http://directory.google.com/Top/Health/Conditions_and_Diseases/**

- Med Help International: **http://www.medhelp.org/HealthTopics/A.html**

- Open Directory Project: **http://dmoz.org/Health/Conditions_and_Diseases/**

- Yahoo.com: **http://dir.yahoo.com/Health/Diseases_and_Conditions/**
- WebMD®Health: **http://my.webmd.com/health_topics**

Finding Associations

There are several Internet directories that provide lists of medical associations with information on or resources relating to Ambien. By consulting all of associations listed in this chapter, you will have nearly exhausted all sources for patient associations concerned with Ambien.

The National Health Information Center (NHIC)

The National Health Information Center (NHIC) offers a free referral service to help people find organizations that provide information about Ambien. For more information, see the NHIC's Web site at **http://www.health.gov/NHIC/** or contact an information specialist by calling 1-800-336-4797.

Directory of Health Organizations

The Directory of Health Organizations, provided by the National Library of Medicine Specialized Information Services, is a comprehensive source of information on associations. The Directory of Health Organizations database can be accessed via the Internet at **http://www.sis.nlm.nih.gov/Dir/DirMain.html**. It is composed of two parts: DIRLINE and Health Hotlines.

The DIRLINE database comprises some 10,000 records of organizations, research centers, and government institutes and associations that primarily focus on health and biomedicine. To access DIRLINE directly, go to the following Web site: **http://dirline.nlm.nih.gov/**. Simply type in "Ambien" (or a synonym), and you will receive information on all relevant organizations listed in the database.

Health Hotlines directs you to toll-free numbers to over 300 organizations. You can access this database directly at **http://www.sis.nlm.nih.gov/hotlines/**. On this page, you are given the option to search by keyword or by browsing the subject list. When you have received your search results, click on the name of the organization for its description and contact information.

The Combined Health Information Database

Another comprehensive source of information on healthcare associations is the Combined Health Information Database. Using the "Detailed Search" option, you will need to limit your search to "Organizations" and "Ambien". Type the following hyperlink into your Web browser: **http://chid.nih.gov/detail/detail.html**. To find associations, use the drop boxes at the bottom of the search page where "You may refine your search by." For publication date, select "All Years." Then, select your preferred language and the format option "Organization Resource Sheet." Type "Ambien" (or synonyms) into the "For these words:"

box. You should check back periodically with this database since it is updated every three months.

The National Organization for Rare Disorders, Inc.

The National Organization for Rare Disorders, Inc. has prepared a Web site that provides, at no charge, lists of associations organized by health topic. You can access this database at the following Web site: **http://www.rarediseases.org/search/orgsearch.html** Type "Ambien" (or a synonym) into the search box, and click "Submit Query."

APPENDIX C. FINDING MEDICAL LIBRARIES

Overview

In this Appendix, we show you how to quickly find a medical library in your area.

Preparation

Your local public library and medical libraries have interlibrary loan programs with the National Library of Medicine (NLM), one of the largest medical collections in the world. According to the NLM, most of the literature in the general and historical collections of the National Library of Medicine is available on interlibrary loan to any library. If you would like to access NLM medical literature, then visit a library in your area that can request the publications for you.[21]

Finding a Local Medical Library

The quickest method to locate medical libraries is to use the Internet-based directory published by the National Network of Libraries of Medicine (NN/LM). This network includes 4626 members and affiliates that provide many services to librarians, health professionals, and the public. To find a library in your area, simply visit http://nnlm.gov/members/adv.html or call 1-800-338-7657.

Medical Libraries in the U.S. and Canada

In addition to the NN/LM, the National Library of Medicine (NLM) lists a number of libraries with reference facilities that are open to the public. The following is the NLM's list and includes hyperlinks to each library's Web site. These Web pages can provide information on hours of operation and other restrictions. The list below is a small sample of

---

[21] Adapted from the NLM: http://www.nlm.nih.gov/psd/cas/interlibrary.html.

libraries recommended by the National Library of Medicine (sorted alphabetically by name of the U.S. state or Canadian province where the library is located)[22]:

- **Alabama:** Health InfoNet of Jefferson County (Jefferson County Library Cooperative, Lister Hill Library of the Health Sciences), **http://www.uab.edu/infonet/**
- **Alabama:** Richard M. Scrushy Library (American Sports Medicine Institute)
- **Arizona:** Samaritan Regional Medical Center: The Learning Center (Samaritan Health System, Phoenix, Arizona), **http://www.samaritan.edu/library/bannerlibs.htm**
- **California:** Kris Kelly Health Information Center (St. Joseph Health System, Humboldt), **http://www.humboldt1.com/~kkhic/index.html**
- **California:** Community Health Library of Los Gatos, **http://www.healthlib.org/orgresources.html**
- **California:** Consumer Health Program and Services (CHIPS) (County of Los Angeles Public Library, Los Angeles County Harbor-UCLA Medical Center Library) - Carson, CA, **http://www.colapublib.org/services/chips.html**
- **California:** Gateway Health Library (Sutter Gould Medical Foundation)
- **California:** Health Library (Stanford University Medical Center), **http://www-med.stanford.edu/healthlibrary/**
- **California:** Patient Education Resource Center - Health Information and Resources (University of California, San Francisco), **http://sfghdean.ucsf.edu/barnett/PERC/default.asp**
- **California:** Redwood Health Library (Petaluma Health Care District), **http://www.phcd.org/rdwdlib.html**
- **California:** Los Gatos PlaneTree Health Library, **http://planetreesanjose.org/**
- **California:** Sutter Resource Library (Sutter Hospitals Foundation, Sacramento), **http://suttermedicalcenter.org/library/**
- **California:** Health Sciences Libraries (University of California, Davis), **http://www.lib.ucdavis.edu/healthsci/**
- **California:** ValleyCare Health Library & Ryan Comer Cancer Resource Center (ValleyCare Health System, Pleasanton), **http://gaelnet.stmarys-ca.edu/other.libs/gbal/east/vchl.html**
- **California:** Washington Community Health Resource Library (Fremont), **http://www.healthlibrary.org/**
- **Colorado:** William V. Gervasini Memorial Library (Exempla Healthcare), **http://www.saintjosephdenver.org/yourhealth/libraries/**
- **Connecticut:** Hartford Hospital Health Science Libraries (Hartford Hospital), **http://www.harthosp.org/library/**
- **Connecticut:** Healthnet: Connecticut Consumer Health Information Center (University of Connecticut Health Center, Lyman Maynard Stowe Library), **http://library.uchc.edu/departm/hnet/**

---

[22] Abstracted from **http://www.nlm.nih.gov/medlineplus/libraries.html**.

- **Connecticut:** Waterbury Hospital Health Center Library (Waterbury Hospital, Waterbury), **http://www.waterburyhospital.com/library/consumer.shtml**
- **Delaware:** Consumer Health Library (Christiana Care Health System, Eugene du Pont Preventive Medicine & Rehabilitation Institute, Wilmington), **http://www.christianacare.org/health_guide/health_guide_pmri_health_info.cfm**
- **Delaware:** Lewis B. Flinn Library (Delaware Academy of Medicine, Wilmington), **http://www.delamed.org/chls.html**
- **Georgia:** Family Resource Library (Medical College of Georgia, Augusta), **http://cmc.mcg.edu/kids_families/fam_resources/fam_res_lib/frl.htm**
- **Georgia:** Health Resource Center (Medical Center of Central Georgia, Macon), **http://www.mccg.org/hrc/hrchome.asp**
- **Hawaii:** Hawaii Medical Library: Consumer Health Information Service (Hawaii Medical Library, Honolulu), **http://hml.org/CHIS/**
- **Idaho:** DeArmond Consumer Health Library (Kootenai Medical Center, Coeur d'Alene), **http://www.nicon.org/DeArmond/index.htm**
- **Illinois:** Health Learning Center of Northwestern Memorial Hospital (Chicago), **http://www.nmh.org/health_info/hlc.html**
- **Illinois:** Medical Library (OSF Saint Francis Medical Center, Peoria), **http://www.osfsaintfrancis.org/general/library/**
- **Kentucky:** Medical Library - Services for Patients, Families, Students & the Public (Central Baptist Hospital, Lexington), **http://www.centralbap.com/education/community/library.cfm**
- **Kentucky:** University of Kentucky - Health Information Library (Chandler Medical Center, Lexington), **http://www.mc.uky.edu/PatientEd/**
- **Louisiana:** Alton Ochsner Medical Foundation Library (Alton Ochsner Medical Foundation, New Orleans), **http://www.ochsner.org/library/**
- **Louisiana:** Louisiana State University Health Sciences Center Medical Library-Shreveport, **http://lib-sh.lsuhsc.edu/**
- **Maine:** Franklin Memorial Hospital Medical Library (Franklin Memorial Hospital, Farmington), **http://www.fchn.org/fmh/lib.htm**
- **Maine:** Gerrish-True Health Sciences Library (Central Maine Medical Center, Lewiston), **http://www.cmmc.org/library/library.html**
- **Maine:** Hadley Parrot Health Science Library (Eastern Maine Healthcare, Bangor), **http://www.emh.org/hll/hpl/guide.htm**
- **Maine:** Maine Medical Center Library (Maine Medical Center, Portland), **http://www.mmc.org/library/**
- **Maine:** Parkview Hospital (Brunswick), **http://www.parkviewhospital.org/**
- **Maine:** Southern Maine Medical Center Health Sciences Library (Southern Maine Medical Center, Biddeford), **http://www.smmc.org/services/service.php3?choice=10**
- **Maine:** Stephens Memorial Hospital's Health Information Library (Western Maine Health, Norway), **http://www.wmhcc.org/Library/**

- **Manitoba, Canada:** Consumer & Patient Health Information Service (University of Manitoba Libraries), http://www.umanitoba.ca/libraries/units/health/reference/chis.html
- **Manitoba, Canada:** J.W. Crane Memorial Library (Deer Lodge Centre, Winnipeg), http://www.deerlodge.mb.ca/crane_library/about.asp
- **Maryland:** Health Information Center at the Wheaton Regional Library (Montgomery County, Dept. of Public Libraries, Wheaton Regional Library), http://www.mont.lib.md.us/healthinfo/hic.asp
- **Massachusetts:** Baystate Medical Center Library (Baystate Health System), http://www.baystatehealth.com/1024/
- **Massachusetts:** Boston University Medical Center Alumni Medical Library (Boston University Medical Center), http://med-libwww.bu.edu/library/lib.html
- **Massachusetts:** Lowell General Hospital Health Sciences Library (Lowell General Hospital, Lowell), http://www.lowellgeneral.org/library/HomePageLinks/WWW.htm
- **Massachusetts:** Paul E. Woodard Health Sciences Library (New England Baptist Hospital, Boston), http://www.nebh.org/health_lib.asp
- **Massachusetts:** St. Luke's Hospital Health Sciences Library (St. Luke's Hospital, Southcoast Health System, New Bedford), http://www.southcoast.org/library/
- **Massachusetts:** Treadwell Library Consumer Health Reference Center (Massachusetts General Hospital), http://www.mgh.harvard.edu/library/chrcindex.html
- **Massachusetts:** UMass HealthNet (University of Massachusetts Medical School, Worchester), http://healthnet.umassmed.edu/
- **Michigan:** Botsford General Hospital Library - Consumer Health (Botsford General Hospital, Library & Internet Services), http://www.botsfordlibrary.org/consumer.htm
- **Michigan:** Helen DeRoy Medical Library (Providence Hospital and Medical Centers), http://www.providence-hospital.org/library/
- **Michigan:** Marquette General Hospital - Consumer Health Library (Marquette General Hospital, Health Information Center), http://www.mgh.org/center.html
- **Michigan:** Patient Education Resouce Center - University of Michigan Cancer Center (University of Michigan Comprehensive Cancer Center, Ann Arbor), http://www.cancer.med.umich.edu/learn/leares.htm
- **Michigan:** Sladen Library & Center for Health Information Resources - Consumer Health Information (Detroit), http://www.henryford.com/body.cfm?id=39330
- **Montana:** Center for Health Information (St. Patrick Hospital and Health Sciences Center, Missoula)
- **National:** Consumer Health Library Directory (Medical Library Association, Consumer and Patient Health Information Section), http://caphis.mlanet.org/directory/index.html
- **National:** National Network of Libraries of Medicine (National Library of Medicine) - provides library services for health professionals in the United States who do not have access to a medical library, http://nnlm.gov/
- **National:** NN/LM List of Libraries Serving the Public (National Network of Libraries of Medicine), http://nnlm.gov/members/

- **Nevada:** Health Science Library, West Charleston Library (Las Vegas-Clark County Library District, Las Vegas), **http://www.lvccld.org/special_collections/medical/index.htm**
- **New Hampshire:** Dartmouth Biomedical Libraries (Dartmouth College Library, Hanover), **http://www.dartmouth.edu/~biomed/resources.htmld/conshealth.htmld/**
- **New Jersey:** Consumer Health Library (Rahway Hospital, Rahway), **http://www.rahwayhospital.com/library.htm**
- **New Jersey:** Dr. Walter Phillips Health Sciences Library (Englewood Hospital and Medical Center, Englewood), **http://www.englewoodhospital.com/links/index.htm**
- **New Jersey:** Meland Foundation (Englewood Hospital and Medical Center, Englewood), **http://www.geocities.com/ResearchTriangle/9360/**
- **New York:** Choices in Health Information (New York Public Library) - NLM Consumer Pilot Project participant, **http://www.nypl.org/branch/health/links.html**
- **New York:** Health Information Center (Upstate Medical University, State University of New York, Syracuse), **http://www.upstate.edu/library/hic/**
- **New York:** Health Sciences Library (Long Island Jewish Medical Center, New Hyde Park), **http://www.lij.edu/library/library.html**
- **New York:** ViaHealth Medical Library (Rochester General Hospital), **http://www.nyam.org/library/**
- **Ohio:** Consumer Health Library (Akron General Medical Center, Medical & Consumer Health Library), **http://www.akrongeneral.org/hwlibrary.htm**
- **Oklahoma:** The Health Information Center at Saint Francis Hospital (Saint Francis Health System, Tulsa), **http://www.sfh-tulsa.com/services/healthinfo.asp**
- **Oregon:** Planetree Health Resource Center (Mid-Columbia Medical Center, The Dalles), **http://www.mcmc.net/phrc/**
- **Pennsylvania:** Community Health Information Library (Milton S. Hershey Medical Center, Hershey), **http://www.hmc.psu.edu/commhealth/**
- **Pennsylvania:** Community Health Resource Library (Geisinger Medical Center, Danville), **http://www.geisinger.edu/education/commlib.shtml**
- **Pennsylvania:** HealthInfo Library (Moses Taylor Hospital, Scranton), **http://www.mth.org/healthwellness.html**
- **Pennsylvania:** Hopwood Library (University of Pittsburgh, Health Sciences Library System, Pittsburgh), **http://www.hsls.pitt.edu/guides/chi/hopwood/index_html**
- **Pennsylvania:** Koop Community Health Information Center (College of Physicians of Philadelphia), **http://www.collphyphil.org/kooppg1.shtml**
- **Pennsylvania:** Learning Resources Center - Medical Library (Susquehanna Health System, Williamsport), **http://www.shscares.org/services/lrc/index.asp**
- **Pennsylvania:** Medical Library (UPMC Health System, Pittsburgh), **http://www.upmc.edu/passavant/library.htm**
- **Quebec, Canada:** Medical Library (Montreal General Hospital), **http://www.mghlib.mcgill.ca/**

- **South Dakota:** Rapid City Regional Hospital Medical Library (Rapid City Regional Hospital), **http://www.rcrh.org/Services/Library/Default.asp**
- **Texas:** Houston HealthWays (Houston Academy of Medicine-Texas Medical Center Library), **http://hhw.library.tmc.edu/**
- **Washington:** Community Health Library (Kittitas Valley Community Hospital), **http://www.kvch.com/**
- **Washington:** Southwest Washington Medical Center Library (Southwest Washington Medical Center, Vancouver), **http://www.swmedicalcenter.com/body.cfm?id=72**

ONLINE GLOSSARIES

The Internet provides access to a number of free-to-use medical dictionaries. The National Library of Medicine has compiled the following list of online dictionaries:

- ADAM Medical Encyclopedia (A.D.A.M., Inc.), comprehensive medical reference:
  http://www.nlm.nih.gov/medlineplus/encyclopedia.html

- MedicineNet.com Medical Dictionary (MedicineNet, Inc.):
  http://www.medterms.com/Script/Main/hp.asp

- Merriam-Webster Medical Dictionary (Inteli-Health, Inc.):
  http://www.intelihealth.com/IH/

- Multilingual Glossary of Technical and Popular Medical Terms in Eight European Languages (European Commission) - Danish, Dutch, English, French, German, Italian, Portuguese, and Spanish: **http://allserv.rug.ac.be/~rvdstich/eugloss/welcome.html**

- On-line Medical Dictionary (CancerWEB): **http://cancerweb.ncl.ac.uk/omd/**

- Rare Diseases Terms (Office of Rare Diseases):
  http://ord.aspensys.com/asp/diseases/diseases.asp

- Technology Glossary (National Library of Medicine) - Health Care Technology:
  http://www.nlm.nih.gov/nichsr/ta101/ta10108.htm

Beyond these, MEDLINEplus contains a very patient-friendly encyclopedia covering every aspect of medicine (licensed from A.D.A.M., Inc.). The ADAM Medical Encyclopedia can be accessed at **http://www.nlm.nih.gov/medlineplus/encyclopedia.html**. ADAM is also available on commercial Web sites such as drkoop.com (**http://www.drkoop.com/**) and Web MD (**http://my.webmd.com/adam/asset/adam_disease_articles/a_to_z/a**).

Online Dictionary Directories

The following are additional online directories compiled by the National Library of Medicine, including a number of specialized medical dictionaries:

- Medical Dictionaries: Medical & Biological (World Health Organization):
  http://www.who.int/hlt/virtuallibrary/English/diction.htm#Medical

- MEL-Michigan Electronic Library List of Online Health and Medical Dictionaries (Michigan Electronic Library): **http://mel.lib.mi.us/health/health-dictionaries.html**

- Patient Education: Glossaries (DMOZ Open Directory Project):
  http://dmoz.org/Health/Education/Patient_Education/Glossaries/

- Web of Online Dictionaries (Bucknell University):
  http://www.yourdictionary.com/diction5.html#medicine

AMBIEN DICTIONARY

The definitions below are derived from official public sources, including the National Institutes of Health [NIH] and the European Union [EU].

5-Hydroxytryptophan: Precursor of serotonin used as antiepileptic and antidepressant. [NIH]

Adrenergic: Activated by, characteristic of, or secreting epinephrine or substances with similar activity; the term is applied to those nerve fibres that liberate norepinephrine at a synapse when a nerve impulse passes, i.e., the sympathetic fibres. [EU]

Adverse Effect: An unwanted side effect of treatment. [NIH]

Affinity: 1. Inherent likeness or relationship. 2. A special attraction for a specific element, organ, or structure. 3. Chemical affinity; the force that binds atoms in molecules; the tendency of substances to combine by chemical reaction. 4. The strength of noncovalent chemical binding between two substances as measured by the dissociation constant of the complex. 5. In immunology, a thermodynamic expression of the strength of interaction between a single antigen-binding site and a single antigenic determinant (and thus of the stereochemical compatibility between them), most accurately applied to interactions among simple, uniform antigenic determinants such as haptens. Expressed as the association constant (K litres mole -1), which, owing to the heterogeneity of affinities in a population of antibody molecules of a given specificity, actually represents an average value (mean intrinsic association constant). 6. The reciprocal of the dissociation constant. [EU]

Agonist: In anatomy, a prime mover. In pharmacology, a drug that has affinity for and stimulates physiologic activity at cell receptors normally stimulated by naturally occurring substances. [EU]

Akathisia: 1. A condition of motor restlessness in which there is a feeling of muscular quivering, an urge to move about constantly, and an inability to sit still, a common extrapyramidal side effect of neuroleptic drugs. 2. An inability to sit down because of intense anxiety at the thought of doing so. [EU]

Alertness: A state of readiness to detect and respond to certain specified small changes occurring at random intervals in the environment. [NIH]

Algorithms: A procedure consisting of a sequence of algebraic formulas and/or logical steps to calculate or determine a given task. [NIH]

Alkaloid: A member of a large group of chemicals that are made by plants and have nitrogen in them. Some alkaloids have been shown to work against cancer. [NIH]

Alpha-1: A protein with the property of inactivating proteolytic enzymes such as leucocyte collagenase and elastase. [NIH]

Alternative medicine: Practices not generally recognized by the medical community as standard or conventional medical approaches and used instead of standard treatments. Alternative medicine includes the taking of dietary supplements, megadose vitamins, and herbal preparations; the drinking of special teas; and practices such as massage therapy, magnet therapy, spiritual healing, and meditation. [NIH]

Amphetamine: A powerful central nervous system stimulant and sympathomimetic. Amphetamine has multiple mechanisms of action including blocking uptake of adrenergics and dopamine, stimulation of release of monamines, and inhibiting monoamine oxidase. Amphetamine is also a drug of abuse and a psychotomimetic. The l- and the d,l-forms are included here. The l-form has less central nervous system activity but stronger cardiovascular effects. The d-form is dextroamphetamine. [NIH]

Anaesthesia: Loss of feeling or sensation. Although the term is used for loss of tactile sensibility, or of any of the other senses, it is applied especially to loss of the sensation of pain, as it is induced to permit performance of surgery or other painful procedures. [EU]

Anaesthetic: 1. Pertaining to, characterized by, or producing anaesthesia. 2. A drug or agent that is used to abolish the sensation of pain. [EU]

Anatomical: Pertaining to anatomy, or to the structure of the organism. [EU]

Anesthesia: A state characterized by loss of feeling or sensation. This depression of nerve function is usually the result of pharmacologic action and is induced to allow performance of surgery or other painful procedures. [NIH]

Anesthetics: Agents that are capable of inducing a total or partial loss of sensation, especially tactile sensation and pain. They may act to induce general anesthesia, in which an unconscious state is achieved, or may act locally to induce numbness or lack of sensation at a targeted site. [NIH]

Antagonism: Interference with, or inhibition of, the growth of a living organism by another living organism, due either to creation of unfavorable conditions (e. g. exhaustion of food supplies) or to production of a specific antibiotic substance (e. g. penicillin). [NIH]

Antiallergic: Counteracting allergy or allergic conditions. [EU]

Anti-Anxiety Agents: Agents that alleviate anxiety, tension, and neurotic symptoms, promote sedation, and have a calming effect without affecting clarity of consciousness or neurologic conditions. Some are also effective as anticonvulsants, muscle relaxants, or anesthesia adjuvants. Adrenergic beta-antagonists are commonly used in the symptomatic treatment of anxiety but are not included here. [NIH]

Antibacterial: A substance that destroys bacteria or suppresses their growth or reproduction. [EU]

Antibiotic: A drug used to treat infections caused by bacteria and other microorganisms. [NIH]

Antibiotic Prophylaxis: Use of antibiotics before, during, or after a diagnostic, therapeutic, or surgical procedure to prevent infectious complications. [NIH]

Anticonvulsant: An agent that prevents or relieves convulsions. [EU]

Antidepressant: A drug used to treat depression. [NIH]

Antidote: A remedy for counteracting a poison. [EU]

Antiemetic: An agent that prevents or alleviates nausea and vomiting. Also antinauseant. [EU]

Antiepileptic: An agent that combats epilepsy. [EU]

Antifungal: Destructive to fungi, or suppressing their reproduction or growth; effective against fungal infections. [EU]

Antipsychotic: Effective in the treatment of psychosis. Antipsychotic drugs (called also neuroleptic drugs and major tranquilizers) are a chemically diverse (including phenothiazines, thioxanthenes, butyrophenones, dibenzoxazepines, dibenzodiazepines, and diphenylbutylpiperidines) but pharmacologically similar class of drugs used to treat schizophrenic, paranoid, schizoaffective, and other psychotic disorders; acute delirium and dementia, and manic episodes (during induction of lithium therapy); to control the movement disorders associated with Huntington's chorea, Gilles de la Tourette's syndrome, and ballismus; and to treat intractable hiccups and severe nausea and vomiting. Antipsychotic agents bind to dopamine, histamine, muscarinic cholinergic, a-adrenergic, and serotonin receptors. Blockade of dopaminergic transmission in various areas is thought to be responsible for their major effects : antipsychotic action by blockade in the mesolimbic and mesocortical areas; extrapyramidal side effects (dystonia, akathisia, parkinsonism, and tardive dyskinesia) by blockade in the basal ganglia; and antiemetic effects by blockade in the chemoreceptor trigger zone of the medulla. Sedation and autonomic side effects (orthostatic hypotension, blurred vision, dry mouth, nasal congestion and constipation) are caused by blockade of histamine, cholinergic, and adrenergic receptors. [EU]

Anxiety: Persistent feeling of dread, apprehension, and impending disaster. [NIH]

Anxiolytic: An anxiolytic or antianxiety agent. [EU]

Aqueous: Having to do with water. [NIH]

Arteries: The vessels carrying blood away from the heart. [NIH]

Aspergillosis: Infections with fungi of the genus Aspergillus. [NIH]

Autonomic: Self-controlling; functionally independent. [EU]

Bacteria: Unicellular prokaryotic microorganisms which generally possess rigid cell walls, multiply by cell division, and exhibit three principal forms: round or coccal, rodlike or bacillary, and spiral or spirochetal. [NIH]

Bactericidal: Substance lethal to bacteria; substance capable of killing bacteria. [NIH]

Barbiturates: A class of chemicals derived from barbituric acid or thiobarbituric acid. Many of these are medically important as sedatives and hypnotics (sedatives, barbiturate), as anesthetics, or as anticonvulsants. [NIH]

Basal Ganglia: Large subcortical nuclear masses derived from the telencephalon and located in the basal regions of the cerebral hemispheres. [NIH]

Base: In chemistry, the nonacid part of a salt; a substance that combines with acids to form salts; a substance that dissociates to give hydroxide ions in aqueous solutions; a substance whose molecule or ion can combine with a proton (hydrogen ion); a substance capable of donating a pair of electrons (to an acid) for the formation of a coordinate covalent bond. [EU]

Benign: Not cancerous; does not invade nearby tissue or spread to other parts of the body. [NIH]

Benzene: Toxic, volatile, flammable liquid hydrocarbon biproduct of coal distillation. It is used as an industrial solvent in paints, varnishes, lacquer thinners, gasoline, etc. Benzene causes central nervous system damage acutely and bone marrow damage chronically and is carcinogenic. It was formerly used as parasiticide. [NIH]

Benzodiazepines: A two-ring heterocyclic compound consisting of a benzene ring fused to a diazepine ring. Permitted is any degree of hydrogenation, any substituents and any H-isomer. [NIH]

Bioavailability: The degree to which a drug or other substance becomes available to the target tissue after administration. [EU]

Biochemical: Relating to biochemistry; characterized by, produced by, or involving chemical reactions in living organisms. [EU]

Biotechnology: Body of knowledge related to the use of organisms, cells or cell-derived constituents for the purpose of developing products which are technically, scientifically and clinically useful. Alteration of biologic function at the molecular level (i.e., genetic engineering) is a central focus; laboratory methods used include transfection and cloning technologies, sequence and structure analysis algorithms, computer databases, and gene and protein structure function analysis and prediction. [NIH]

Biphasic: Having two phases; having both a sporophytic and a gametophytic phase in the life cycle. [EU]

Bladder: The organ that stores urine. [NIH]

Blastomycosis: A fungal infection that may appear in two forms: 1) a primary lesion characterized by the formation of a small cutaneous nodule and small nodules along the lymphatics that may heal within several months; and 2) chronic granulomatous lesions characterized by thick crusts, warty growths, and unusual vascularity and infection in the middle or upper lobes of the lung. [NIH]

Blood Platelets: Non-nucleated disk-shaped cells formed in the megakaryocyte and found in the blood of all mammals. They are mainly involved in blood coagulation. [NIH]

Blood pressure: The pressure of blood against the walls of a blood vessel or heart chamber. Unless there is reference to another location, such as the pulmonary artery or one of the heart chambers, it refers to the pressure in the systemic arteries, as measured, for example, in the forearm. [NIH]

Blood vessel: A tube in the body through which blood circulates. Blood vessels include a network of arteries, arterioles, capillaries, venules, and veins. [NIH]

Branch: Most commonly used for branches of nerves, but applied also to other structures. [NIH]

Buspirone: An anxiolytic agent and a serotonin receptor agonist belonging to the azaspirodecanedione class of compounds. Its structure is unrelated to those of the benzodiazepines, but it has an efficacy comparable to diazepam. [NIH]

Caffeine: A methylxanthine naturally occurring in some beverages and also used as a pharmacological agent. Caffeine's most notable pharmacological effect is as a central nervous system stimulant, increasing alertness and producing agitation. It also relaxes smooth muscle, stimulates cardiac muscle, stimulates diuresis, and appears to be useful in the treatment of some types of headache. Several cellular actions of caffeine have been observed, but it is not entirely clear how each contributes to its pharmacological profile. Among the most important are inhibition of cyclic nucleotide phosphodiesterases, antagonism of adenosine receptors, and modulation of intracellular calcium handling. [NIH]

Calcium: A basic element found in nearly all organized tissues. It is a member of the alkaline earth family of metals with the atomic symbol Ca, atomic number 20, and atomic weight 40. Calcium is the most abundant mineral in the body and combines with phosphorus to form calcium phosphate in the bones and teeth. It is essential for the normal functioning of nerves and muscles and plays a role in blood coagulation (as factor IV) and in many enzymatic processes. [NIH]

Candidiasis: Infection with a fungus of the genus Candida. It is usually a superficial infection of the moist cutaneous areas of the body, and is generally caused by C. albicans; it most commonly involves the skin (dermatocandidiasis), oral mucous membranes (thrush, def. 1), respiratory tract (bronchocandidiasis), and vagina (vaginitis). Rarely there is a systemic infection or endocarditis. Called also moniliasis, candidosis, oidiomycosis, and formerly blastodendriosis. [EU]

Capsules: Hard or soft soluble containers used for the oral administration of medicine. [NIH]

Cardiac: Having to do with the heart. [NIH]

Cardiovascular: Having to do with the heart and blood vessels. [NIH]

Case report: A detailed report of the diagnosis, treatment, and follow-up of an individual patient. Case reports also contain some demographic information about the patient (for example, age, gender, ethnic origin). [NIH]

Case series: A group or series of case reports involving patients who were given similar treatment. Reports of case series usually contain detailed information about the individual patients. This includes demographic information (for example, age, gender, ethnic origin) and information on diagnosis, treatment, response to treatment, and follow-up after treatment. [NIH]

Cell: The individual unit that makes up all of the tissues of the body. All living things are made up of one or more cells. [NIH]

Central Nervous System: The main information-processing organs of the nervous system, consisting of the brain, spinal cord, and meninges. [NIH]

Central Nervous System Infections: Pathogenic infections of the brain, spinal cord, and meninges. DNA virus infections; RNA virus infections; bacterial infections; mycoplasma infections; Spirochaetales infections; fungal infections; protozoan infections; helminthiasis; and prion diseases may involve the central nervous system as a primary or secondary process. [NIH]

Cerebral: Of or pertaining of the cerebrum or the brain. [EU]

Cerebrum: The largest part of the brain. It is divided into two hemispheres, or halves, called the cerebral hemispheres. The cerebrum controls muscle functions of the body and also controls speech, emotions, reading, writing, and learning. [NIH]

Chemoreceptor: A receptor adapted for excitation by chemical substances, e.g., olfactory and gustatory receptors, or a sense organ, as the carotid body or the aortic (supracardial) bodies, which is sensitive to chemical changes in the blood stream, especially reduced oxygen content, and reflexly increases both respiration and blood pressure. [EU]

Chlordiazepoxide: An anxiolytic benzodiazepine derivative with anticonvulsant, sedative, and amnesic properties. It has also been used in the symptomatic treatment of alcohol withdrawl. [NIH]

Cholinergic: Resembling acetylcholine in pharmacological action; stimulated by or releasing acetylcholine or a related compound. [EU]

Chorea: Involuntary, forcible, rapid, jerky movements that may be subtle or become confluent, markedly altering normal patterns of movement. Hypotonia and pendular reflexes are often associated. Conditions which feature recurrent or persistent episodes of chorea as a primary manifestation of disease are referred to as choreatic disorders. Chorea is also a frequent manifestation of basal ganglia diseases. [NIH]

Chronic: A disease or condition that persists or progresses over a long period of time. [NIH]

Clinical trial: A research study that tests how well new medical treatments or other interventions work in people. Each study is designed to test new methods of screening, prevention, diagnosis, or treatment of a disease. [NIH]

Cloning: The production of a number of genetically identical individuals; in genetic engineering, a process for the efficient replication of a great number of identical DNA molecules. [NIH]

Coca: Any of several South American shrubs of the Erythroxylon genus (and family) that yield cocaine; the leaves are chewed with alum for CNS stimulation. [NIH]

Cocaine: An alkaloid ester extracted from the leaves of plants including coca. It is a local anesthetic and vasoconstrictor and is clinically used for that purpose, particularly in the eye, ear, nose, and throat. It also has powerful central nervous system effects similar to the amphetamines and is a drug of abuse. Cocaine, like amphetamines, acts by multiple mechanisms on brain catecholaminergic neurons; the mechanism of its reinforcing effects is thought to involve inhibition of dopamine uptake. [NIH]

Comatose: Pertaining to or affected with coma. [EU]

Complement: A term originally used to refer to the heat-labile factor in serum that causes immune cytolysis, the lysis of antibody-coated cells, and now referring to the entire functionally related system comprising at least 20 distinct serum proteins that is the effector not only of immune cytolysis but also of other biologic functions. Complement activation occurs by two different sequences, the classic and alternative pathways. The proteins of the classic pathway are termed 'components of complement' and are designated by the symbols C1 through C9. C1 is a calcium-dependent complex of three distinct proteins C1q, C1r and C1s. The proteins of the alternative pathway (collectively referred to as the properdin system) and complement regulatory proteins are known by semisystematic or trivial names. Fragments resulting from proteolytic cleavage of complement proteins are designated with lower-case letter suffixes, e.g., C3a. Inactivated fragments may be designated with the suffix 'i', e.g. C3bi. Activated components or complexes with biological activity are designated by a bar over the symbol e.g. C1 or C4b,2a. The classic pathway is activated by the binding of C1 to classic pathway activators, primarily antigen-antibody complexes containing IgM, IgG1, IgG3; C1q binds to a single IgM molecule or two adjacent IgG molecules. The alternative pathway can be activated by IgA immune complexes and also by nonimmunologic materials including bacterial endotoxins, microbial polysaccharides, and cell walls. Activation of the classic pathway triggers an enzymatic cascade involving C1, C4, C2 and C3; activation of the alternative pathway triggers a cascade involving C3 and factors B, D and P. Both result in the cleavage of C5 and the formation of the membrane attack complex. Complement activation also results in the formation of many biologically active complement fragments that act as anaphylatoxins, opsonins, or chemotactic factors. [EU]

Complementary and alternative medicine: CAM. Forms of treatment that are used in addition to (complementary) or instead of (alternative) standard treatments. These practices are not considered standard medical approaches. CAM includes dietary supplements, megadose vitamins, herbal preparations, special teas, massage therapy, magnet therapy, spiritual healing, and meditation. [NIH]

Complementary medicine: Practices not generally recognized by the medical community as standard or conventional medical approaches and used to enhance or complement the standard treatments. Complementary medicine includes the taking of dietary supplements, megadose vitamins, and herbal preparations; the drinking of special teas; and practices such as massage therapy, magnet therapy, spiritual healing, and meditation. [NIH]

Computational Biology: A field of biology concerned with the development of techniques for the collection and manipulation of biological data, and the use of such data to make biological discoveries or predictions. This field encompasses all computational methods and theories applicable to molecular biology and areas of computer-based techniques for solving biological problems including manipulation of models and datasets. [NIH]

Conception: The onset of pregnancy, marked by implantation of the blastocyst; the formation of a viable zygote. [EU]

Congestion: Excessive or abnormal accumulation of blood in a part. [EU]

Conjugated: Acting or operating as if joined; simultaneous. [EU]

Consciousness: Sense of awareness of self and of the environment. [NIH]

Constipation: Infrequent or difficult evacuation of feces. [NIH]

Consumption: Pulmonary tuberculosis. [NIH]

Contraceptive: An agent that diminishes the likelihood of or prevents conception. [EU]

Contraindications: Any factor or sign that it is unwise to pursue a certain kind of action or treatment, e. g. giving a general anesthetic to a person with pneumonia. [NIH]

Controlled study: An experiment or clinical trial that includes a comparison (control) group.

[NIH]

Coordination: Muscular or motor regulation or the harmonious cooperation of muscles or groups of muscles, in a complex action or series of actions. [NIH]

Coronary: Encircling in the manner of a crown; a term applied to vessels; nerves, ligaments, etc. The term usually denotes the arteries that supply the heart muscle and, by extension, a pathologic involvement of them. [EU]

Coronary Thrombosis: Presence of a thrombus in a coronary artery, often causing a myocardial infarction. [NIH]

Cortex: The outer layer of an organ or other body structure, as distinguished from the internal substance. [EU]

Cortical: Pertaining to or of the nature of a cortex or bark. [EU]

Cranial: Pertaining to the cranium, or to the anterior (in animals) or superior (in humans) end of the body. [EU]

Craniocerebral Trauma: Traumatic injuries involving the cranium and intracranial structures (i.e., brain; cranial nerves; meninges; and other structures). Injuries may be classified by whether or not the skull is penetrated (i.e., penetrating vs. nonpenetrating) or whether there is an associated hemorrhage. [NIH]

Crystallization: The formation of crystals; conversion to a crystalline form. [EU]

Curare: Plant extracts from several species, including Strychnos toxifera, S. castelnaei, S. crevauxii, and Chondodendron tomentosum, that produce paralysis of skeletal muscle and are used adjunctively with general anesthesia. These extracts are toxic and must be used with the administration of artificial respiration. [NIH]

Curative: Tending to overcome disease and promote recovery. [EU]

Cyclic: Pertaining to or occurring in a cycle or cycles; the term is applied to chemical compounds that contain a ring of atoms in the nucleus. [EU]

Cytochrome: Any electron transfer hemoprotein having a mode of action in which the transfer of a single electron is effected by a reversible valence change of the central iron atom of the heme prosthetic group between the +2 and +3 oxidation states; classified as cytochromes a in which the heme contains a formyl side chain, cytochromes b, which contain protoheme or a closely similar heme that is not covalently bound to the protein, cytochromes c in which protoheme or other heme is covalently bound to the protein, and cytochromes d in which the iron-tetrapyrrole has fewer conjugated double bonds than the hemes have. Well-known cytochromes have been numbered consecutively within groups and are designated by subscripts (beginning with no subscript), e.g. cytochromes c, c1, C2, . New cytochromes are named according to the wavelength in nanometres of the absorption maximum of the a-band of the iron (II) form in pyridine, e.g., c-555. [EU]

Databases, Bibliographic: Extensive collections, reputedly complete, of references and citations to books, articles, publications, etc., generally on a single subject or specialized subject area. Databases can operate through automated files, libraries, or computer disks. The concept should be differentiated from factual databases which is used for collections of data and facts apart from bibliographic references to them. [NIH]

Deletion: A genetic rearrangement through loss of segments of DNA (chromosomes), bringing sequences, which are normally separated, into close proximity. [NIH]

Delirium: (DSM III-R) an acute, reversible organic mental disorder characterized by reduced ability to maintain attention to external stimuli and disorganized thinking as manifested by rambling, irrelevant, or incoherent speech; there are also a reduced level of consciousness, sensory misperceptions, disturbance of the sleep-wakefulness cycle and level of psychomotor activity, disorientation to time, place, or person, and memory impairment Delirium may be caused by a large number of conditions resulting in derangement of cerebral metabolism, including systemic infection, poisoning, drug intoxication or withdrawal, seizures or head trauma, and metabolic disturbances such as hypoxia, hypoglycaemia, fluid, electrolyte, or acid-base imbalances, or hepatic or renal failure. Called also acute confusional state and acute brain syndrome. [EU]

Dementia: An acquired organic mental disorder with loss of intellectual abilities of sufficient severity to interfere with social or occupational functioning. The dysfunction is multifaceted and involves memory, behavior, personality, judgment, attention, spatial relations, language, abstract thought, and other executive functions. The intellectual decline is usually progressive, and initially spares the level of consciousness. [NIH]

Dendrites: Extensions of the nerve cell body. They are short and branched and receive stimuli from other neurons. [NIH]

Dextroamphetamine: The d-form of amphetamine. It is a central nervous system stimulant and a sympathomimetic. It has also been used in the treatment of narcolepsy and of attention deficit disorders and hyperactivity in children. Dextroamphetamine has multiple mechanisms of action including blocking uptake of adrenergics and dopamine, stimulating release of monamines, and inhibiting monoamine oxidase. It is also a drug of abuse and a psychotomimetic. [NIH]

Diagnostic procedure: A method used to identify a disease. [NIH]

Direct: 1. Straight; in a straight line. 2. Performed immediately and without the intervention of subsidiary means. [EU]

Discrimination: The act of qualitative and/or quantitative differentiation between two or more stimuli. [NIH]

Disinfectant: An agent that disinfects; applied particularly to agents used on inanimate objects. [EU]

Disorientation: The loss of proper bearings, or a state of mental confusion as to time, place, or identity. [EU]

Distal: Remote; farther from any point of reference; opposed to proximal. In dentistry, used to designate a position on the dental arch farther from the median line of the jaw. [EU]

Diuresis: Increased excretion of urine. [EU]

Dopamine: An endogenous catecholamine and prominent neurotransmitter in several systems of the brain. In the synthesis of catecholamines from tyrosine, it is the immediate precursor to norepinephrine and epinephrine. Dopamine is a major transmitter in the extrapyramidal system of the brain, and important in regulating movement. A family of dopaminergic receptor subtypes mediate its action. Dopamine is used pharmacologically for its direct (beta adrenergic agonist) and indirect (adrenergic releasing) sympathomimetic effects including its actions as an inotropic agent and as a renal vasodilator. [NIH]

Dosage Forms: Completed forms of the pharmaceutical preparation in which prescribed doses of medication are included. They are designed to resist action by gastric fluids, prevent vomiting and nausea, reduce or alleviate the undesirable taste and smells associated with oral administration, achieve a high concentration of drug at target site, or produce a delayed or long-acting drug effect. They include capsules, liniments, ointments, pharmaceutical solutions, powders, tablets, etc. [NIH]

Dose-dependent: Refers to the effects of treatment with a drug. If the effects change when the dose of the drug is changed, the effects are said to be dose dependent. [NIH]

Drug Interactions: The action of a drug that may affect the activity, metabolism, or toxicity of another drug. [NIH]

Drug Tolerance: Progressive diminution of the susceptibility of a human or animal to the effects of a drug, resulting from its continued administration. It should be differentiated from drug resistance wherein an organism, disease, or tissue fails to respond to the intended effectiveness of a chemical or drug. It should also be differentiated from maximum tolerated dose and no-observed-adverse-effect level. [NIH]

Dyskinesia: Impairment of the power of voluntary movement, resulting in fragmentary or incomplete movements. [EU]

Dystonia: Disordered tonicity of muscle. [EU]

Efficacy: The extent to which a specific intervention, procedure, regimen, or service produces a beneficial result under ideal conditions. Ideally, the determination of efficacy is based on the results of a randomized control trial. [NIH]

Elective: Subject to the choice or decision of the patient or physician; applied to procedures that are advantageous to the patient but not urgent. [EU]

Electrolyte: A substance that dissociates into ions when fused or in solution, and thus becomes capable of conducting electricity; an ionic solute. [EU]

Electrons: Stable elementary particles having the smallest known negative charge, present in all elements; also called negatrons. Positively charged electrons are called positrons. The numbers, energies and arrangement of electrons around atomic nuclei determine the chemical identities of elements. Beams of electrons are called cathode rays or beta rays, the latter being a high-energy biproduct of nuclear decay. [NIH]

Environmental Health: The science of controlling or modifying those conditions, influences, or forces surrounding man which relate to promoting, establishing, and maintaining health. [NIH]

Enzymes: Biological molecules that possess catalytic activity. They may occur naturally or be synthetically created. Enzymes are usually proteins, however catalytic RNA and catalytic DNA molecules have also been identified. [NIH]

Ethanol: A clear, colorless liquid rapidly absorbed from the gastrointestinal tract and distributed throughout the body. It has bactericidal activity and is used often as a topical disinfectant. It is widely used as a solvent and preservative in pharmaceutical preparations as well as serving as the primary ingredient in alcoholic beverages. [NIH]

Evoke: The electric response recorded from the cerebral cortex after stimulation of a peripheral sense organ. [NIH]

Extrapyramidal: Outside of the pyramidal tracts. [EU]

Family Planning: Programs or services designed to assist the family in controlling reproduction by either improving or diminishing fertility. [NIH]

Femoral: Pertaining to the femur, or to the thigh. [EU]

Femoral Neck Fractures: Fractures of the short, constricted portion of the thigh bone between the femur head and the trochanters. It excludes intertrochanteric fractures which are hip fractures. [NIH]

Femur: The longest and largest bone of the skeleton, it is situated between the hip and the knee. [NIH]

Fixation: 1. The act or operation of holding, suturing, or fastening in a fixed position. 2. The condition of being held in a fixed position. 3. In psychiatry, a term with two related but distinct meanings : (1) arrest of development at a particular stage, which like regression (return to an earlier stage), if temporary is a normal reaction to setbacks and difficulties but if protracted or frequent is a cause of developmental failures and emotional problems, and (2) a close and suffocating attachment to another person, especially a childhood figure, such as one's mother or father. Both meanings are derived from psychoanalytic theory and refer to 'fixation' of libidinal energy either in a specific erogenous zone, hence fixation at the oral, anal, or phallic stage, or in a specific object, hence mother or father fixation. 4. The use of a fixative (q.v.) to preserve histological or cytological specimens. 5. In chemistry, the process whereby a substance is removed from the gaseous or solution phase and localized, as in carbon dioxide fixation or nitrogen fixation. 6. In ophthalmology, direction of the gaze so that the visual image of the object falls on the fovea centralis. 7. In film processing, the chemical removal of all undeveloped salts of the film emulsion, leaving only the developed silver to form a permanent image. [EU]

Fluconazole: Triazole antifungal agent that is used to treat oropharyngeal candidiasis and cryptococcal meningitis in AIDS. [NIH]

Flumazenil: A potent benzodiazepine receptor antagonist. Since it reverses the sedative and other actions of benzodiazepines, it has been suggested as an antidote to benzodiazepine overdoses. [NIH]

Flunitrazepam: Benzodiazepine with pharmacologic actions similar to those of diazepam. The United States Government has banned the importation of this drug. Steps are being taken to reclassify this substance as a Schedule 1 drug with no accepted medical use. [NIH]

Fluorescence: The property of emitting radiation while being irradiated. The radiation emitted is usually of longer wavelength than that incident or absorbed, e.g., a substance can be irradiated with invisible radiation and emit visible light. X-ray fluorescence is used in diagnosis. [NIH]

Fluoxetine: The first highly specific serotonin uptake inhibitor. It is used as an antidepressant and often has a more acceptable side-effects profile than traditional antidepressants. [NIH]

Fraud: Exploitation through misrepresentation of the facts or concealment of the purposes of the exploiter. [NIH]

Ganglia: Clusters of multipolar neurons surrounded by a capsule of loosely organized connective tissue located outside the central nervous system. [NIH]

Gas: Air that comes from normal breakdown of food. The gases are passed out of the body through the rectum (flatus) or the mouth (burp). [NIH]

Gas exchange: Primary function of the lungs; transfer of oxygen from inhaled air into the blood and of carbon dioxide from the blood into the lungs. [NIH]

Gastric: Having to do with the stomach. [NIH]

Gastrointestinal: Refers to the stomach and intestines. [NIH]

Gastrointestinal tract: The stomach and intestines. [NIH]

Gene: The functional and physical unit of heredity passed from parent to offspring. Genes are pieces of DNA, and most genes contain the information for making a specific protein. [NIH]

Gland: An organ that produces and releases one or more substances for use in the body. Some glands produce fluids that affect tissues or organs. Others produce hormones or participate in blood production. [NIH]

Glycoprotein: A protein that has sugar molecules attached to it. [NIH]

Governing Board: The group in which legal authority is vested for the control of health-related institutions and organizations. [NIH]

Half-Life: The time it takes for a substance (drug, radioactive nuclide, or other) to lose half of its pharmacologic, physiologic, or radiologic activity. [NIH]

Headache: Pain in the cranial region that may occur as an isolated and benign symptom or as a manifestation of a wide variety of conditions including subarachnoid hemorrhage; craniocerebral trauma; central nervous system infections; intracranial hypertension; and other disorders. In general, recurrent headaches that are not associated with a primary disease process are referred to as headache disorders (e.g., migraine). [NIH]

Headache Disorders: Common conditions characterized by persistent or recurrent headaches. Headache syndrome classification systems may be based on etiology (e.g., vascular headache, post-traumatic headaches, etc.), temporal pattern (e.g., cluster headache, paroxysmal hemicrania, etc.), and precipitating factors (e.g., cough headache). [NIH]

Heme: The color-furnishing portion of hemoglobin. It is found free in tissues and as the prosthetic group in many hemeproteins. [NIH]

Hemorrhage: Bleeding or escape of blood from a vessel. [NIH]

Hemostasis: The process which spontaneously arrests the flow of blood from vessels carrying blood under pressure. It is accomplished by contraction of the vessels, adhesion and aggregation of formed blood elements, and the process of blood or plasma coagulation. [NIH]

Hepatic: Refers to the liver. [NIH]

Hip Fractures: Fractures of the femur head, the femur neck, the trochanters, or the inter- or subtrochanteric region. Excludes fractures of the acetabulum and fractures of the femoral shaft below the subtrochanteric region. For the fractures of the femur neck the specific term femoral neck fractures is available. [NIH]

Histamine: 1H-Imidazole-4-ethanamine. A depressor amine derived by enzymatic decarboxylation of histidine. It is a powerful stimulant of gastric secretion, a constrictor of bronchial smooth muscle, a vasodilator, and also a centrally acting neurotransmitter. [NIH]

Hydrogen: The first chemical element in the periodic table. It has the atomic symbol H, atomic number 1, and atomic weight 1. It exists, under normal conditions, as a colorless, odorless, tasteless, diatomic gas. Hydrogen ions are protons. Besides the common H1 isotope, hydrogen exists as the stable isotope deuterium and the unstable, radioactive isotope tritium. [NIH]

Hypertension: Persistently high arterial blood pressure. Currently accepted threshold levels are 140 mm Hg systolic and 90 mm Hg diastolic pressure. [NIH]

Hypnotic: A drug that acts to induce sleep. [EU]

Hypoglycaemia: An abnormally diminished concentration of glucose in the blood, which may lead to tremulousness, cold sweat, piloerection, hypothermia, and headache, accompanied by irritability, confusion, hallucinations, bizarre behaviour, and ultimately, convulsions and coma. [EU]

Hypokinesia: Slow or diminished movement of body musculature. It may be associated with basal ganglia diseases; mental disorders; prolonged inactivity due to illness; experimental protocols used to evaluate the physiologic effects of immobility; and other conditions. [NIH]

Hypotension: Abnormally low blood pressure. [NIH]

Hypoxia: Reduction of oxygen supply to tissue below physiological levels despite adequate perfusion of the tissue by blood. [EU]

Id: The part of the personality structure which harbors the unconscious instinctive desires and strivings of the individual. [NIH]

Immune system: The organs, cells, and molecules responsible for the recognition and disposal of foreign ("non-self") material which enters the body. [NIH]

Impairment: In the context of health experience, an impairment is any loss or abnormality of psychological, physiological, or anatomical structure or function. [NIH]

In vitro: In the laboratory (outside the body). The opposite of in vivo (in the body). [NIH]

In vivo: In the body. The opposite of in vitro (outside the body or in the laboratory). [NIH]

Indicative: That indicates; that points out more or less exactly; that reveals fairly clearly. [EU]

Induction: The act or process of inducing or causing to occur, especially the production of a specific morphogenetic effect in the developing embryo through the influence of evocators or organizers, or the production of anaesthesia or unconsciousness by use of appropriate agents. [EU]

Infarction: A pathological process consisting of a sudden insufficient blood supply to an area, which results in necrosis of that area. It is usually caused by a thrombus, an embolus, or a vascular torsion. [NIH]

Infection: 1. Invasion and multiplication of microorganisms in body tissues, which may be clinically unapparent or result in local cellular injury due to competitive metabolism, toxins, intracellular replication, or antigen-antibody response. The infection may remain localized, subclinical, and temporary if the body's defensive mechanisms are effective. A local infection may persist and spread by extension to become an acute, subacute, or chronic clinical infection or disease state. A local infection may also become systemic when the microorganisms gain access to the lymphatic or vascular system. 2. An infectious disease. [EU]

Infusion: A method of putting fluids, including drugs, into the bloodstream. Also called intravenous infusion. [NIH]

Ingestion: Taking into the body by mouth [NIH]

Insomnia: Difficulty in going to sleep or getting enough sleep. [NIH]

Intermittent: Occurring at separated intervals; having periods of cessation of activity. [EU]

Intoxication: Poisoning, the state of being poisoned. [EU]

Intracellular: Inside a cell. [NIH]

Intravenous: IV. Into a vein. [NIH]

Ions: An atom or group of atoms that have a positive or negative electric charge due to a gain (negative charge) or loss (positive charge) of one or more electrons. Atoms with a positive charge are known as cations; those with a negative charge are anions. [NIH]

Itraconazole: An antifungal agent that has been used in the treatment of histoplasmosis, blastomycosis, cryptococcal meningitis, and aspergillosis. [NIH]

Jet lag: Symptoms produced in human beings by fast travel through large meridian difference. [NIH]

Kb: A measure of the length of DNA fragments, 1 Kb = 1000 base pairs. The largest DNA fragments are up to 50 kilobases long. [NIH]

Ketoconazole: Broad spectrum antifungal agent used for long periods at high doses, especially in immunosuppressed patients. [NIH]

Kinetics: The study of rate dynamics in chemical or physical systems. [NIH]

Lag: The time elapsing between application of a stimulus and the resulting reaction. [NIH]

Latency: The period of apparent inactivity between the time when a stimulus is presented and the moment a response occurs. [NIH]

Leucocyte: All the white cells of the blood and their precursors (myeloid cell series, lymphoid cell series) but commonly used to indicate granulocytes exclusive of lymphocytes. [NIH]

Library Services: Services offered to the library user. They include reference and circulation. [NIH]

Life cycle: The successive stages through which an organism passes from fertilized ovum or spore to the fertilized ovum or spore of the next generation. [NIH]

Lithium: An element in the alkali metals family. It has the atomic symbol Li, atomic number 3, and atomic weight 6.94. Salts of lithium are used in treating manic-depressive disorders. [NIH]

Lorazepam: An anti-anxiety agent with few side effects. It also has hypnotic, anticonvulsant, and considerable sedative properties and has been proposed as a preanesthetic agent. [NIH]

Manic: Affected with mania. [EU]

Mediator: An object or substance by which something is mediated, such as (1) a structure of the nervous system that transmits impulses eliciting a specific response; (2) a chemical substance (transmitter substance) that induces activity in an excitable tissue, such as nerve or muscle; or (3) a substance released from cells as the result of the interaction of antigen with antibody or by the action of antigen with a sensitized lymphocyte. [EU]

MEDLINE: An online database of MEDLARS, the computerized bibliographic Medical Literature Analysis and Retrieval System of the National Library of Medicine. [NIH]

Membranes: Thin layers of tissue which cover parts of the body, separate adjacent cavities, or connect adjacent structures. [NIH]

Memory: Complex mental function having four distinct phases: (1) memorizing or learning, (2) retention, (3) recall, and (4) recognition. Clinically, it is usually subdivided into immediate, recent, and remote memory. [NIH]

Meningitis: Inflammation of the meninges. When it affects the dura mater, the disease is termed pachymeningitis; when the arachnoid and pia mater are involved, it is called leptomeningitis, or meningitis proper. [EU]

Mesolimbic: Inner brain region governing emotion and drives. [NIH]

Metabolite: Any substance produced by metabolism or by a metabolic process. [EU]

Methanol: A colorless, flammable liquid used in the manufacture of formaldehyde and acetic acid, in chemical synthesis, antifreeze, and as a solvent. Ingestion of methanol is toxic and may cause blindness. [NIH]

Methohexital: An intravenous anesthetic with a short duration of action that may be used for induction of anesthesia. [NIH]

Methylphenidate: A central nervous system stimulant used most commonly in the treatment of attention-deficit disorders in children and for narcolepsy. Its mechanisms appear to be similar to those of dextroamphetamine. [NIH]

MI: Myocardial infarction. Gross necrosis of the myocardium as a result of interruption of the blood supply to the area; it is almost always caused by atherosclerosis of the coronary arteries, upon which coronary thrombosis is usually superimposed. [NIH]

Molecular: Of, pertaining to, or composed of molecules : a very small mass of matter. [EU]

Molecule: A chemical made up of two or more atoms. The atoms in a molecule can be the same (an oxygen molecule has two oxygen atoms) or different (a water molecule has two hydrogen atoms and one oxygen atom). Biological molecules, such as proteins and DNA, can be made up of many thousands of atoms. [NIH]

Monoamine: Enzyme that breaks down dopamine in the astrocytes and microglia. [NIH]

Motility: The ability to move spontaneously. [EU]

Motion Sickness: Sickness caused by motion, as sea sickness, train sickness, car sickness, and air sickness. [NIH]

Motor Activity: The physical activity of an organism as a behavioral phenomenon. [NIH]

Motor nerve: An efferent nerve conveying an impulse that excites muscular contraction. [NIH]

Movement Disorders: Syndromes which feature dyskinesias as a cardinal manifestation of the disease process. Included in this category are degenerative, hereditary, post-infectious, medication-induced, post-inflammatory, and post-traumatic conditions. [NIH]

Muscle relaxant: An agent that specifically aids in reducing muscle tension, as those acting at the polysynaptic neurons of motor nerves (e.g. meprobamate) or at the myoneural junction (curare and related compounds). [EU]

Muscle tension: A force in a material tending to produce extension; the state of being stretched. [NIH]

Myocardium: The muscle tissue of the heart composed of striated, involuntary muscle known as cardiac muscle. [NIH]

Naive: Used to describe an individual who has never taken a certain drug or class of drugs (e. g., AZT-naive, antiretroviral-naive), or to refer to an undifferentiated immune system cell. [NIH]

Narcolepsy: A condition of unknown cause characterized by a periodic uncontrollable tendency to fall asleep. [NIH]

Nausea: An unpleasant sensation in the stomach usually accompanied by the urge to vomit. Common causes are early pregnancy, sea and motion sickness, emotional stress, intense pain, food poisoning, and various enteroviruses. [NIH]

Necrosis: A pathological process caused by the progressive degradative action of enzymes that is generally associated with severe cellular trauma. It is characterized by mitochondrial swelling, nuclear flocculation, uncontrolled cell lysis, and ultimately cell death. [NIH]

Need: A state of tension or dissatisfaction felt by an individual that impels him to action toward a goal he believes will satisfy the impulse. [NIH]

Nerve: A cordlike structure of nervous tissue that connects parts of the nervous system with other tissues of the body and conveys nervous impulses to, or away from, these tissues. [NIH]

Nervous System: The entire nerve apparatus composed of the brain, spinal cord, nerves and ganglia. [NIH]

Neuroanatomy: Study of the anatomy of the nervous system as a specialty or discipline. [NIH]

Neuroleptic: A term coined to refer to the effects on cognition and behaviour of antipsychotic drugs, which produce a state of apathy, lack of initiative, and limited range of emotion and in psychotic patients cause a reduction in confusion and agitation and normalization of psychomotor activity. [EU]

Neurons: The basic cellular units of nervous tissue. Each neuron consists of a body, an axon, and dendrites. Their purpose is to receive, conduct, and transmit impulses in the nervous system. [NIH]

Neuropathy: A problem in any part of the nervous system except the brain and spinal cord. Neuropathies can be caused by infection, toxic substances, or disease. [NIH]

Neurosis: Functional derangement due to disorders of the nervous system which does not affect the psychic personality of the patient. [NIH]

Neurotic: 1. Pertaining to or characterized by neurosis. 2. A person affected with a neurosis. [EU]

Ocular: 1. Of, pertaining to, or affecting the eye. 2. Eyepiece. [EU]

Ointments: Semisolid preparations used topically for protective emollient effects or as a vehicle for local administration of medications. Ointment bases are various mixtures of fats, waxes, animal and plant oils and solid and liquid hydrocarbons. [NIH]

Orthostatic: Pertaining to or caused by standing erect. [EU]

Outpatient: A patient who is not an inmate of a hospital but receives diagnosis or treatment in a clinic or dispensary connected with the hospital. [NIH]

Overdose: An accidental or deliberate dose of a medication or street drug that is in excess of what is normally used. [NIH]

Oxidation: The act of oxidizing or state of being oxidized. Chemically it consists in the increase of positive charges on an atom or the loss of negative charges. Most biological oxidations are accomplished by the removal of a pair of hydrogen atoms (dehydrogenation) from a molecule. Such oxidations must be accompanied by reduction of an acceptor molecule. Univalent o. indicates loss of one electron; divalent o., the loss of two electrons. [EU]

Palliative: 1. Affording relief, but not cure. 2. An alleviating medicine. [EU]

Palsy: Disease of the peripheral nervous system occurring usually after many years of increased lead absorption. [NIH]

Parkinsonism: A group of neurological disorders characterized by hypokinesia, tremor, and muscular rigidity. [EU]

Perfusion: Bathing an organ or tissue with a fluid. In regional perfusion, a specific area of the body (usually an arm or a leg) receives high doses of anticancer drugs through a blood vessel. Such a procedure is performed to treat cancer that has not spread. [NIH]

Peripheral Nervous System: The nervous system outside of the brain and spinal cord. The peripheral nervous system has autonomic and somatic divisions. The autonomic nervous system includes the enteric, parasympathetic, and sympathetic subdivisions. The somatic nervous system includes the cranial and spinal nerves and their ganglia and the peripheral sensory receptors. [NIH]

Peripheral Neuropathy: Nerve damage, usually affecting the feet and legs; causing pain, numbness, or a tingling feeling. Also called "somatic neuropathy" or "distal sensory polyneuropathy." [NIH]

Peroral: Performed through or administered through the mouth. [EU]

Pharmaceutical Solutions: Homogeneous liquid preparations that contain one or more chemical substances dissolved, i.e., molecularly dispersed, in a suitable solvent or mixture of mutually miscible solvents. For reasons of their ingredients, method of preparation, or use, they do not fall into another group of products. [NIH]

Pharmacodynamic: Is concerned with the response of living tissues to chemical stimuli, that is, the action of drugs on the living organism in the absence of disease. [NIH]

Pharmacokinetic: The mathematical analysis of the time courses of absorption, distribution, and elimination of drugs. [NIH]

Pharmacologic: Pertaining to pharmacology or to the properties and reactions of drugs. [EU]

Physiologic: Having to do with the functions of the body. When used in the phrase "physiologic age," it refers to an age assigned by general health, as opposed to calendar age.

[NIH]

Plants: Multicellular, eukaryotic life forms of the kingdom Plantae. They are characterized by a mainly photosynthetic mode of nutrition; essentially unlimited growth at localized regions of cell divisions (meristems); cellulose within cells providing rigidity; the absence of organs of locomotion; absense of nervous and sensory systems; and an alteration of haploid and diploid generations. [NIH]

Plasma: The clear, yellowish, fluid part of the blood that carries the blood cells. The proteins that form blood clots are in plasma. [NIH]

Poisoning: A condition or physical state produced by the ingestion, injection or inhalation of, or exposure to a deleterious agent. [NIH]

Practice Guidelines: Directions or principles presenting current or future rules of policy for the health care practitioner to assist him in patient care decisions regarding diagnosis, therapy, or related clinical circumstances. The guidelines may be developed by government agencies at any level, institutions, professional societies, governing boards, or by the convening of expert panels. The guidelines form a basis for the evaluation of all aspects of health care and delivery. [NIH]

Premedication: Preliminary administration of a drug preceding a diagnostic, therapeutic, or surgical procedure. The commonest types of premedication are antibiotics (antibiotic prophylaxis) and anti-anxiety agents. It does not include preanesthetic medication. [NIH]

Progeny: The offspring produced in any generation. [NIH]

Progressive: Advancing; going forward; going from bad to worse; increasing in scope or severity. [EU]

Promethazine: A phenothiazine derivative with histamine H1-blocking, antimuscarinic, and sedative properties. It is used as an antiallergic, in pruritus, for motion sickness and sedation, and also in animals. [NIH]

Protease: Proteinase (= any enzyme that catalyses the splitting of interior peptide bonds in a protein). [EU]

Protein S: The vitamin K-dependent cofactor of activated protein C. Together with protein C, it inhibits the action of factors VIIIa and Va. A deficiency in protein S can lead to recurrent venous and arterial thrombosis. [NIH]

Proteins: Polymers of amino acids linked by peptide bonds. The specific sequence of amino acids determines the shape and function of the protein. [NIH]

Proteolytic: 1. Pertaining to, characterized by, or promoting proteolysis. 2. An enzyme that promotes proteolysis (= the splitting of proteins by hydrolysis of the peptide bonds with formation of smaller polypeptides). [EU]

Pruritus: An intense itching sensation that produces the urge to rub or scratch the skin to obtain relief. [NIH]

Psychiatric: Pertaining to or within the purview of psychiatry. [EU]

Psychic: Pertaining to the psyche or to the mind; mental. [EU]

Psychomotor: Pertaining to motor effects of cerebral or psychic activity. [EU]

Psychomotor Performance: The coordination of a sensory or ideational (cognitive) process and a motor activity. [NIH]

Psychosis: A mental disorder characterized by gross impairment in reality testing as evidenced by delusions, hallucinations, markedly incoherent speech, or disorganized and agitated behaviour without apparent awareness on the part of the patient of the incomprehensibility of his behaviour; the term is also used in a more general sense to refer to mental disorders in which mental functioning is sufficiently impaired as to interfere grossly with the patient's capacity to meet the ordinary demands of life. Historically, the term has been applied to many conditions, e.g. manic-depressive psychosis, that were first described in psychotic patients, although many patients with the disorder are not judged psychotic. [EU]

Psychotomimetic: Psychosis miming. [NIH]

Public Policy: A course or method of action selected, usually by a government, from among alternatives to guide and determine present and future decisions. [NIH]

Publishing: "The business or profession of the commercial production and issuance of literature" (Webster's 3d). It includes the publisher, publication processes, editing and editors. Production may be by conventional printing methods or by electronic publishing. [NIH]

Radiation: Emission or propagation of electromagnetic energy (waves/rays), or the waves/rays themselves; a stream of electromagnetic particles (electrons, neutrons, protons, alpha particles) or a mixture of these. The most common source is the sun. [NIH]

Radioactive: Giving off radiation. [NIH]

Randomized: Describes an experiment or clinical trial in which animal or human subjects are assigned by chance to separate groups that compare different treatments. [NIH]

Receptor: A molecule inside or on the surface of a cell that binds to a specific substance and causes a specific physiologic effect in the cell. [NIH]

Receptors, Serotonin: Cell-surface proteins that bind serotonin and trigger intracellular changes which influence the behavior of cells. Several types of serotonin receptors have been recognized which differ in their pharmacology, molecular biology, and mode of action. [NIH]

Recombinant: A cell or an individual with a new combination of genes not found together in either parent; usually applied to linked genes. [EU]

Refer: To send or direct for treatment, aid, information, de decision. [NIH]

Refraction: A test to determine the best eyeglasses or contact lenses to correct a refractive error (myopia, hyperopia, or astigmatism). [NIH]

Regimen: A treatment plan that specifies the dosage, the schedule, and the duration of treatment. [NIH]

Relaxant: 1. Lessening or reducing tension. 2. An agent that lessens tension. [EU]

Renal failure: Progressive renal insufficiency and uremia, due to irreversible and progressive renal glomerular tubular or interstitial disease. [NIH]

Respiratory failure: Inability of the lungs to conduct gas exchange. [NIH]

Response rate: The percentage of patients whose cancer shrinks or disappears after treatment. [NIH]

Restless legs: Legs characterized by or showing inability to remain at rest. [EU]

Rigidity: Stiffness or inflexibility, chiefly that which is abnormal or morbid; rigor. [EU]

Ritonavir: An HIV protease inhibitor that works by interfering with the reproductive cycle of HIV. [NIH]

Saccades: An abrupt voluntary shift in ocular fixation from one point to another, as occurs in reading. [NIH]

Schizoid: Having qualities resembling those found in greater degree in schizophrenics; a person of schizoid personality. [NIH]

Schizophrenia: A mental disorder characterized by a special type of disintegration of the personality. [NIH]

Schizotypal Personality Disorder: A personality disorder in which there are oddities of thought (magical thinking, paranoid ideation, suspiciousness), perception (illusions, depersonalization), speech (digressive, vague, overelaborate), and behavior (inappropriate affect in social interactions, frequently social isolation) that are not severe enough to characterize schizophrenia. [NIH]

Screening: Checking for disease when there are no symptoms. [NIH]

Sedative: 1. Allaying activity and excitement. 2. An agent that allays excitement. [EU]

Sedatives, Barbiturate: Those derivatives of barbituric or thiobarbituric acid that are used as hypnotics or sedatives. The structural class of all such derivatives, regardless of use, is barbiturates. [NIH]

Seizures: Clinical or subclinical disturbances of cortical function due to a sudden, abnormal, excessive, and disorganized discharge of brain cells. Clinical manifestations include abnormal motor, sensory and psychic phenomena. Recurrent seizures are usually referred to as epilepsy or "seizure disorder." [NIH]

Serotonin: A biochemical messenger and regulator, synthesized from the essential amino acid L-tryptophan. In humans it is found primarily in the central nervous system, gastrointestinal tract, and blood platelets. Serotonin mediates several important physiological functions including neurotransmission, gastrointestinal motility, hemostasis, and cardiovascular integrity. Multiple receptor families (receptors, serotonin) explain the broad physiological actions and distribution of this biochemical mediator. [NIH]

Sertraline: A selective serotonin uptake inhibitor that is used in the treatment of depression. [NIH]

Side effect: A consequence other than the one(s) for which an agent or measure is used, as the adverse effects produced by a drug, especially on a tissue or organ system other than the one sought to be benefited by its administration. [EU]

Sleep Deprivation: The state of being deprived of sleep under experimental conditions, due to life events, or from a wide variety of pathophysiologic causes such as medication effect, chronic illness, psychiatric illness, or sleep disorder. [NIH]

Smooth muscle: Muscle that performs automatic tasks, such as constricting blood vessels. [NIH]

Solvent: 1. Dissolving; effecting a solution. 2. A liquid that dissolves or that is capable of dissolving; the component of a solution that is present in greater amount. [EU]

Somatic: 1. Pertaining to or characteristic of the soma or body. 2. Pertaining to the body wall in contrast to the viscera. [EU]

Somnambulism: A parasomnia characterized by a partial arousal that occurs during stage IV of non-REM sleep. Affected individuals exhibit semipurposeful behaviors such as ambulation and are difficult to fully awaken. Children are primarily affected, with a peak age range of 4-6 years. [NIH]

Specialist: In medicine, one who concentrates on 1 special branch of medical science. [NIH]

Spectrum: A charted band of wavelengths of electromagnetic vibrations obtained by refraction and diffraction. By extension, a measurable range of activity, such as the range of bacteria affected by an antibiotic (antibacterial s.) or the complete range of manifestations of a disease. [EU]

Spinal cord: The main trunk or bundle of nerves running down the spine through holes in the spinal bone (the vertebrae) from the brain to the level of the lower back. [NIH]

Stimulant: 1. Producing stimulation; especially producing stimulation by causing tension on muscle fibre through the nervous tissue. 2. An agent or remedy that produces stimulation. [EU]

Stimulus: That which can elicit or evoke action (response) in a muscle, nerve, gland or other excitable issue, or cause an augmenting action upon any function or metabolic process. [NIH]

Stress: Forcibly exerted influence; pressure. Any condition or situation that causes strain or tension. Stress may be either physical or psychologic, or both. [NIH]

Subarachnoid: Situated or occurring between the arachnoid and the pia mater. [EU]

Subclinical: Without clinical manifestations; said of the early stage(s) of an infection or other disease or abnormality before symptoms and signs become apparent or detectable by clinical examination or laboratory tests, or of a very mild form of an infection or other disease or abnormality. [EU]

Subcutaneous: Beneath the skin. [NIH]

Substance P: An eleven-amino acid neurotransmitter that appears in both the central and peripheral nervous systems. It is involved in transmission of pain, causes rapid contractions of the gastrointestinal smooth muscle, and modulates inflammatory and immune responses. [NIH]

Subtrochanteric: Below a trochanter. [NIH]

Sympathomimetic: 1. Mimicking the effects of impulses conveyed by adrenergic postganglionic fibres of the sympathetic nervous system. 2. An agent that produces effects similar to those of impulses conveyed by adrenergic postganglionic fibres of the sympathetic nervous system. Called also adrenergic. [EU]

Symptomatic: Having to do with symptoms, which are signs of a condition or disease. [NIH]

Symptomatic treatment: Therapy that eases symptoms without addressing the cause of disease. [NIH]

Systemic: Affecting the entire body. [NIH]

Tardive: Marked by lateness, late; said of a disease in which the characteristic lesion is late in appearing. [EU]

Therapeutics: The branch of medicine which is concerned with the treatment of diseases, palliative or curative. [NIH]

Tin: A trace element that is required in bone formation. It has the atomic symbol Sn, atomic number 50, and atomic weight 118.71. [NIH]

Tissue: A group or layer of cells that are alike in type and work together to perform a specific function. [NIH]

Tolerance: 1. The ability to endure unusually large doses of a drug or toxin. 2. Acquired drug tolerance; a decreasing response to repeated constant doses of a drug or the need for increasing doses to maintain a constant response. [EU]

Tonicity: The normal state of muscular tension. [NIH]

Topical: On the surface of the body. [NIH]

Toxic: Having to do with poison or something harmful to the body. Toxic substances usually cause unwanted side effects. [NIH]

Toxicity: The quality of being poisonous, especially the degree of virulence of a toxic microbe or of a poison. [EU]

Toxicology: The science concerned with the detection, chemical composition, and pharmacologic action of toxic substances or poisons and the treatment and prevention of toxic manifestations. [NIH]

Transfection: The uptake of naked or purified DNA into cells, usually eukaryotic. It is analogous to bacterial transformation. [NIH]

Trauma: Any injury, wound, or shock, must frequently physical or structural shock, producing a disturbance. [NIH]

Tremor: Cyclical movement of a body part that can represent either a physiologic process or a manifestation of disease. Intention or action tremor, a common manifestation of cerebellar diseases, is aggravated by movement. In contrast, resting tremor is maximal when there is no attempt at voluntary movement, and occurs as a relatively frequent manifestation of Parkinson disease. [NIH]

Triazolam: A short-acting benzodiazepine used in the treatment of insomnia. Some countries temporarily withdrew triazolam from the market because of concerns about adverse reactions, mostly psychological, associated with higher dose ranges. Its use at lower doses with appropriate care and labeling has been reaffirmed by the FDA and most other countries. [NIH]

Trigger zone: Dolorogenic zone (= producing or causing pain). [EU]

Tryptophan: An essential amino acid that is necessary for normal growth in infants and for nitrogen balance in adults. It is a precursor serotonin and niacin. [NIH]

Tuberculosis: Any of the infectious diseases of man and other animals caused by species of Mycobacterium. [NIH]

Unconscious: Experience which was once conscious, but was subsequently rejected, as the "personal unconscious". [NIH]

Urethra: The tube through which urine leaves the body. It empties urine from the bladder. [NIH]

Urine: Fluid containing water and waste products. Urine is made by the kidneys, stored in the bladder, and leaves the body through the urethra. [NIH]

Vascular: Pertaining to blood vessels or indicative of a copious blood supply. [EU]

Vein: Vessel-carrying blood from various parts of the body to the heart. [NIH]

Venlafaxine: An antidepressant drug that is being evaluated for the treatment of hot flashes in women who have breast cancer. [NIH]

Veterinary Medicine: The medical science concerned with the prevention, diagnosis, and treatment of diseases in animals. [NIH]

Visual Perception: The selecting and organizing of visual stimuli based on the individual's past experience. [NIH]

Vitro: Descriptive of an event or enzyme reaction under experimental investigation occurring outside a living organism. Parts of an organism or microorganism are used together with artificial substrates and/or conditions. [NIH]

Vivo: Outside of or removed from the body of a living organism. [NIH]

Wakefulness: A state in which there is an enhanced potential for sensitivity and an efficient responsiveness to external stimuli. [NIH]

Withdrawal: 1. A pathological retreat from interpersonal contact and social involvement, as may occur in schizophrenia, depression, or schizoid avoidant and schizotypal personality disorders. 2. (DSM III-R) A substance-specific organic brain syndrome that follows the cessation of use or reduction in intake of a psychoactive substance that had been regularly used to induce a state of intoxication. [EU]

INDEX

5
5-Hydroxytryptophan, 29, 63
A
Adrenergic, 63, 64, 70, 81
Adverse Effect, 63, 80
Affinity, 63
Agonist, 22, 63, 66, 70
Akathisia, 63, 65
Alertness, 63, 66
Algorithms, 63, 65
Alkaloid, 63, 67
Alpha-1, 4, 23, 63
Alternative medicine, 36, 63
Amphetamine, 23, 63, 70
Anaesthesia, 64, 74
Anaesthetic, 16, 64
Anatomical, 64, 74
Anesthesia, 64, 69, 75
Anesthetics, 64, 65
Antagonism, 64, 66
Antiallergic, 64, 78
Anti-Anxiety Agents, 64, 78
Antibacterial, 64, 80
Antibiotic, 64, 78, 80
Antibiotic Prophylaxis, 64, 78
Anticonvulsant, 64, 67, 75
Antidepressant, 63, 64, 72, 82
Antidote, 64, 72
Antiemetic, 64, 65
Antiepileptic, 63, 64
Antifungal, 64, 72, 74
Antipsychotic, 17, 64, 76
Anxiety, 63, 64, 65, 75
Anxiolytic, 65, 66, 67
Aqueous, 22, 65
Arteries, 65, 66, 69, 75
Aspergillosis, 65, 74
Autonomic, 65, 77
B
Bacteria, 64, 65, 80
Bactericidal, 65, 71
Barbiturates, 4, 65, 80
Basal Ganglia, 65, 67, 73
Base, 32, 33, 65, 70, 74
Benign, 65, 73
Benzene, 65
Benzodiazepines, 3, 7, 12, 23, 27, 34, 65, 66, 72

Bioavailability, 32, 65
Biochemical, 65, 80
Biotechnology, 5, 36, 47, 65
Biphasic, 32, 65
Bladder, 66, 82
Blastomycosis, 66, 74
Blood Platelets, 66, 80
Blood pressure, 66, 67, 73
Blood vessel, 66, 77, 80, 82
Branch, 59, 66, 80, 81
Buspirone, 12, 66
C
Caffeine, 10, 16, 22, 23, 66
Calcium, 66, 68
Candidiasis, 66, 72
Capsules, 66, 70
Cardiac, 66, 76
Cardiovascular, 14, 64, 66, 80
Case report, 6, 9, 19, 27, 66
Case series, 16, 66
Cell, 63, 65, 67, 68, 70, 74, 75, 76, 78, 79
Central Nervous System, 63, 65, 66, 67, 70, 72, 73, 75, 80
Central Nervous System Infections, 67, 73
Cerebral, 22, 23, 65, 67, 70, 71, 78
Cerebrum, 67
Chemoreceptor, 65, 67
Chlordiazepoxide, 4, 67
Cholinergic, 64, 67
Chorea, 64, 67
Chronic, 6, 9, 19, 22, 36, 66, 67, 74, 80
Clinical trial, 4, 47, 67, 68, 79
Cloning, 65, 67
Coca, 67
Cocaine, 23, 67
Comatose, 6, 27, 67
Complement, 68
Complementary and alternative medicine, 27, 30, 68
Complementary medicine, 27, 68
Computational Biology, 47, 68
Conception, 68
Congestion, 65, 68
Conjugated, 68, 69
Consciousness, 64, 68, 69, 70
Constipation, 65, 68
Consumption, 22, 68
Contraceptive, 18, 68

Contraindications, ii, 68
Controlled study, 6, 15, 68
Coordination, 69, 78
Coronary, 69, 75
Coronary Thrombosis, 69, 75
Cortex, 23, 69, 71
Cortical, 69, 80
Cranial, 69, 73, 77
Craniocerebral Trauma, 69, 73
Crystallization, 33, 69
Curare, 69, 76
Curative, 69, 81
Cyclic, 66, 69
Cytochrome, 10, 69

D
Databases, Bibliographic, 47, 69
Deletion, 23, 69
Delirium, 9, 19, 64, 69
Dementia, 7, 64, 70
Dendrites, 70, 76
Dextroamphetamine, 64, 70, 75
Diagnostic procedure, 31, 36, 70
Direct, iii, 39, 70, 79
Discrimination, 18, 24, 70
Disinfectant, 70, 71
Disorientation, 70
Distal, 70, 77
Diuresis, 66, 70
Dopamine, 63, 64, 67, 70, 76
Dosage Forms, 32, 33, 70
Dose-dependent, 4, 70
Drug Interactions, 7, 40, 70
Drug Tolerance, 71, 81
Dyskinesia, 14, 65, 71
Dystonia, 17, 65, 71

E
Efficacy, 19, 66, 71
Elective, 13, 71
Electrolyte, 70, 71
Electrons, 65, 71, 74, 77, 79
Environmental Health, 46, 48, 71
Enzymes, 63, 71, 76
Ethanol, 9, 71
Evoke, 71, 81
Extrapyramidal, 63, 65, 70, 71

F
Family Planning, 47, 71
Femoral, 71, 73
Femoral Neck Fractures, 71, 73
Femur, 71, 73
Fixation, 71, 79
Fluconazole, 11, 72

Flumazenil, 9, 22, 72
Flunitrazepam, 11, 13, 72
Fluorescence, 15, 72
Fluoxetine, 12, 15, 72
Fraud, 16, 72

G
Ganglia, 72, 76, 77
Gas, 72, 73, 79
Gas exchange, 72, 79
Gastric, 70, 72, 73
Gastrointestinal, 71, 72, 80, 81
Gastrointestinal tract, 71, 72, 80
Gene, 65, 72
Gland, 72, 81
Glycoprotein, 10, 72
Governing Board, 72, 78

H
Half-Life, 32, 73
Headache, 19, 66, 73
Headache Disorders, 73
Heme, 69, 73
Hemorrhage, 69, 73
Hemostasis, 73, 80
Hepatic, 70, 73
Hip Fractures, 18, 71, 73
Histamine, 64, 73, 78
Hydrogen, 65, 73, 75, 77
Hypertension, 73
Hypnotic, 8, 27, 32, 33, 73, 75
Hypoglycaemia, 70, 73
Hypokinesia, 73, 77
Hypotension, 14, 65, 73
Hypoxia, 70, 73

I
Id, 25, 28, 52, 58, 60, 73
Immune system, 74, 76
Impairment, 10, 16, 24, 70, 71, 74, 78
In vitro, 18, 74
In vivo, 18, 74
Indicative, 74, 82
Induction, 64, 74, 75
Infarction, 69, 74, 75
Infection, 66, 70, 74, 76, 81
Infusion, 9, 74
Ingestion, 7, 22, 74, 75, 78
Insomnia, 3, 6, 9, 11, 12, 15, 17, 19, 22, 27, 28, 29, 33, 36, 74, 82
Intermittent, 11, 74
Intoxication, 11, 70, 74, 82
Intracellular, 66, 74, 79
Intravenous, 23, 74, 75
Ions, 65, 71, 73, 74

Itraconazole, 10, 11, 74
J
Jet lag, 10, 22, 74
K
Kb, 46, 74
Ketoconazole, 11, 74
Kinetics, 7, 8, 32, 74
L
Lag, 74
Latency, 8, 34, 74
Leucocyte, 63, 75
Library Services, 58, 75
Life cycle, 66, 75
Lithium, 64, 75
Lorazepam, 4, 75
M
Manic, 64, 75, 79
Mediator, 75, 80
MEDLINE, 47, 75
Membranes, 23, 66, 75
Memory, 8, 10, 13, 14, 15, 70, 75
Meningitis, 72, 74, 75
Mesolimbic, 65, 75
Metabolite, 8, 75
Methanol, 33, 75
Methohexital, 4, 75
Methylphenidate, 13, 75
MI, 61, 75
Molecular, 12, 47, 49, 65, 68, 75, 79
Molecule, 65, 68, 75, 77, 79
Monoamine, 63, 70, 76
Motility, 76, 80
Motion Sickness, 76, 78
Motor Activity, 11, 76, 78
Motor nerve, 76
Movement Disorders, 14, 64, 76
Muscle relaxant, 3, 64, 76
Muscle tension, 76
Myocardium, 75, 76
N
Naive, 23, 76
Narcolepsy, 70, 75, 76
Nausea, 64, 70, 76
Necrosis, 74, 75, 76
Need, 3, 41, 53, 76, 81
Nerve, 63, 64, 70, 75, 76, 77, 81
Nervous System, 7, 63, 67, 75, 76, 77, 81
Neuroanatomy, 28, 76
Neuroleptic, 63, 64, 76
Neurons, 23, 67, 70, 72, 76
Neuropathy, 76, 77
Neurosis, 76, 77

Neurotic, 12, 64, 77
O
Ocular, 13, 77, 79
Ointments, 70, 77
Orthostatic, 14, 65, 77
Outpatient, 9, 22, 77
Overdose, 6, 77
Oxidation, 69, 77
P
Palliative, 77, 81
Palsy, 17, 77
Parkinsonism, 17, 65, 77
Perfusion, 22, 73, 77
Peripheral Nervous System, 77, 81
Peripheral Neuropathy, 3, 77
Peroral, 33, 77
Pharmaceutical Solutions, 70, 77
Pharmacodynamic, 12, 32, 77
Pharmacokinetic, 12, 18, 32, 77
Pharmacologic, 27, 64, 72, 73, 77, 81
Physiologic, 63, 73, 77, 79, 82
Plants, 63, 67, 78
Plasma, 15, 32, 73, 78
Poisoning, 70, 74, 76, 78
Practice Guidelines, 48, 78
Premedication, 27, 78
Progeny, 23, 78
Progressive, 17, 70, 71, 76, 78, 79
Promethazine, 16, 78
Protease, 78, 79
Protein S, 65, 78
Proteins, 68, 71, 75, 78, 79
Proteolytic, 63, 68, 78
Pruritus, 78
Psychiatric, 17, 78, 80
Psychic, 77, 78, 80
Psychomotor, 8, 13, 14, 15, 70, 76, 78
Psychomotor Performance, 8, 13, 14, 78
Psychosis, 64, 78, 79
Psychotomimetic, 63, 70, 79
Public Policy, 47, 79
Publishing, 5, 79
R
Radiation, 72, 79
Radioactive, 73, 79
Randomized, 6, 9, 22, 71, 79
Receptor, 4, 8, 14, 22, 23, 24, 66, 67, 70, 72, 79, 80
Receptors, Serotonin, 79, 80
Recombinant, 14, 79
Refer, 1, 68, 72, 76, 78, 79
Refraction, 79, 80

Regimen, 71, 79
Relaxant, 79
Renal failure, 70, 79
Respiratory failure, 6, 79
Response rate, 4, 79
Restless legs, 18, 24, 79
Rigidity, 77, 78, 79
Ritonavir, 10, 79

S
Saccades, 13, 79
Schizoid, 79, 82
Schizophrenia, 79, 80, 82
Schizotypal Personality Disorder, 80, 82
Screening, 67, 80
Sedative, 67, 72, 75, 78, 80
Sedatives, Barbiturate, 65, 80
Seizures, 6, 13, 19, 70, 80
Serotonin, 15, 19, 63, 65, 66, 72, 79, 80, 82
Sertraline, 7, 80
Side effect, 7, 39, 41, 63, 65, 75, 80, 81
Sleep Deprivation, 28, 80
Smooth muscle, 66, 73, 80, 81
Solvent, 65, 71, 75, 77, 80
Somatic, 77, 80
Somnambulism, 18, 80
Specialist, 53, 80
Spectrum, 9, 74, 80
Spinal cord, 67, 76, 77, 80
Stimulant, 63, 66, 70, 73, 75, 80
Stimulus, 10, 22, 74, 81
Stress, 12, 23, 76, 81
Subarachnoid, 73, 81
Subclinical, 74, 80, 81
Subcutaneous, 23, 81
Substance P, 75, 81
Subtrochanteric, 73, 81
Sympathomimetic, 63, 70, 81

Symptomatic, 64, 67, 81
Symptomatic treatment, 64, 67, 81
Systemic, 40, 66, 70, 74, 81

T
Tardive, 65, 81
Therapeutics, 7, 8, 11, 12, 34, 40, 81
Tin, 77, 81
Tissue, 18, 65, 71, 72, 73, 75, 76, 77, 80, 81
Tolerance, 13, 24, 34, 81
Tonicity, 71, 81
Topical, 71, 81
Toxic, iv, 65, 69, 75, 76, 81
Toxicity, 70, 81
Toxicology, 6, 9, 12, 16, 18, 19, 23, 48, 81
Transfection, 65, 82
Trauma, 70, 76, 82
Tremor, 77, 82
Triazolam, 4, 6, 8, 9, 10, 15, 18, 22, 23, 82
Trigger zone, 65, 82
Tryptophan, 80, 82
Tuberculosis, 68, 82

U
Unconscious, 64, 73, 82
Urethra, 82
Urine, 12, 66, 70, 82

V
Vascular, 19, 73, 74, 82
Vein, 74, 82
Venlafaxine, 13, 82
Veterinary Medicine, 47, 82
Visual Perception, 19, 82
Vitro, 82
Vivo, 82

W
Wakefulness, 69, 82
Withdrawal, 6, 24, 70, 82

88 Ambien